Contents

Theme	Unit		Page
	How to use this book		
SELF AND INTERPERSONAL RELATIONSHIPS	1	I Can Be Anything!	4
	2	Making Decisions	6
	3	Understanding Feelings	8
	4	Family Relationships	10
	5	Building Relationships	12
	6	Special Feelings	14
	7	I Am Changing	16
	8	Dealing with Changes	18
	9	I Can Control Myself	20
	10	Communication	22
	11	Drugs	24
	12	Beautiful People	26
SEXUALITY AND SEXUAL HEALTH	1	Growing Up	28
	2	Alike but Different	30
	3	Good Touch, Bad Touch	32
	4	HIV Prevention	34
	5	Caring For People with HIV and AIDS	36
EATING AND FITNESS	1	Fruit and Vegetables	38
	2	Healthy Food Choices	40
	3	Safe Food	42
	4	Muscles and Movement	44
	5	Safe Exercise and Competition	46
	6	Eating and Fitness Choices	48
MANAGING THE ENVIRONMENT	1	Our Environment	50
	2	Trees and Forests	52
	3	Pollution	54
	4	Put It in the Bin!	56
	5	Improving Our Environment	58
	6	Reduce, Reuse, Recycle	60
	7	Finding Things Out	62

SELF AND INTERPERSONAL RELATIONSHIPS

1 I Can Be Anything!

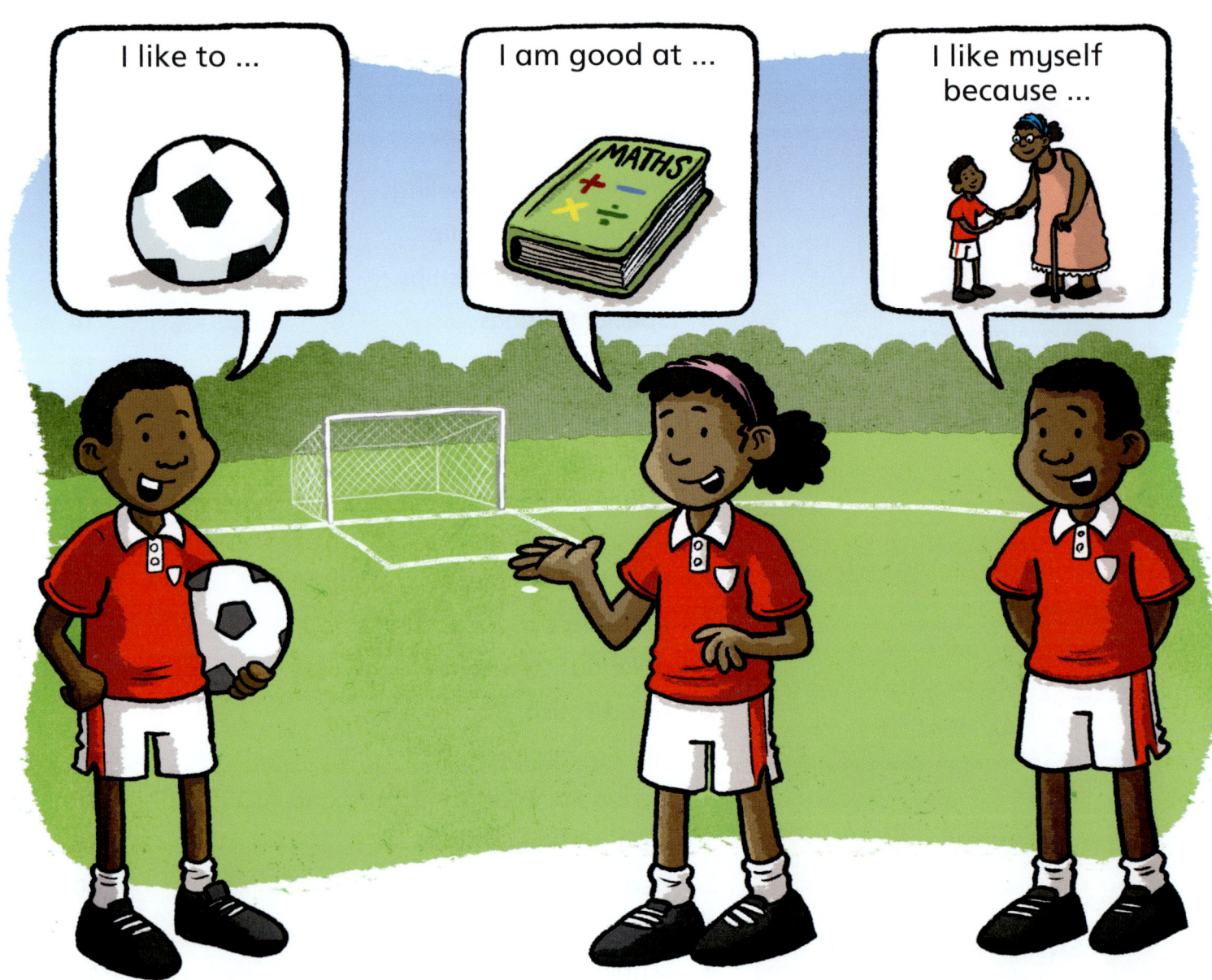

Activity 1

Share with your partner:
1 Two things you like to do.
2 Three things you are good at (talents).
3 Two things you like about yourself.

▶ Key Life Skills: **Self-awareness**, Creative thinking, Decision-making

Student's Book 2

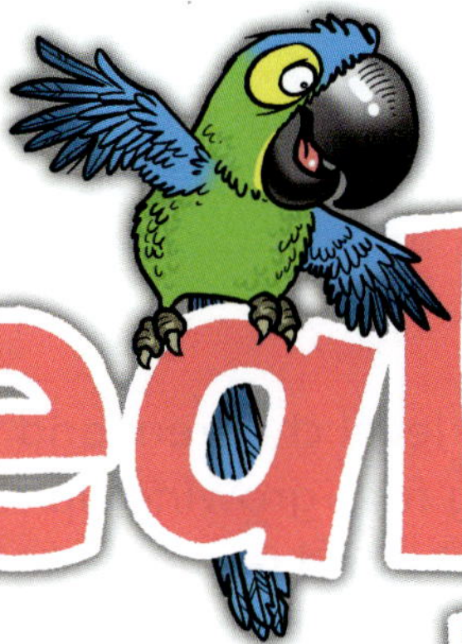

Health and Family Life Education

for primary level

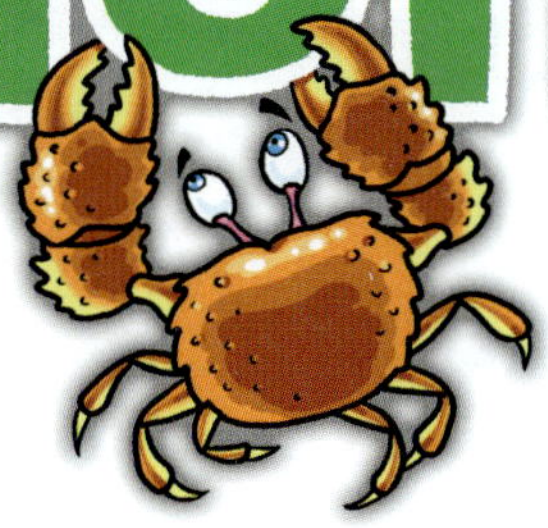

Author and advisor team:

Fortuna Anthony • Jenelle Babb • Pauline Bain • Hermione Baptiste • Vindra Cassie

Gerard Drakes • Clare Eastland • Mavis Fuller • Janice Ho Lung • Sharlene Johnson

Elaine King • Louise Lawrence-Rose • Nordia McIntosh-Vassell • Heather Richards

Glenda Rolle • Gina Sanguinetti Phillips • Rebecca Tortello • Esther Utoh • Pat Warner

macmillan education

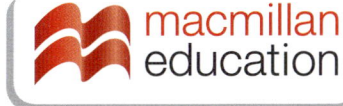

How to use this book

Macmillan's HFLE course addresses the needs of primary level children, and those of their teachers and parents, to help them cope with the challenges they face growing up today. This lower primary Student's Book will help young children to understand and manage themselves and their surroundings in an age-appropriate way. It emphasises the learning of life skills and covers the relevant parts of the CARICOM Regional Curriculum Framework for ages 5 to 12 years.

You will find the four CARICOM themes: **Self and Interpersonal Relationships**, **Sexuality and Sexual Health**, **Eating and Fitness** and **Managing the Environment**, all colour-coded for easy reference.

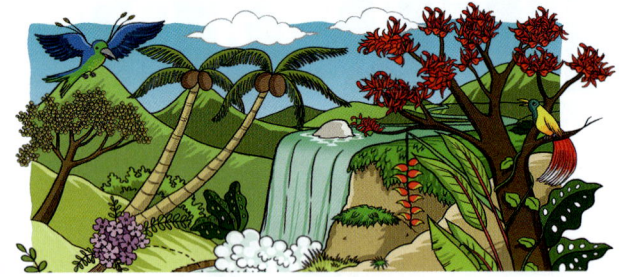

The sky is blue. The hills are green.
The river and sea are clear and clean.

Look at and discuss the pictures. Ask questions to guide thinking.

Read the text to, or with, the children.

Relate the pictures and text to the children's own experiences. Encourage children to reflect upon and talk about their own feelings and actions.

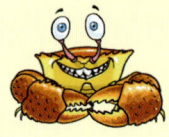 Our friendly crab and parrot icons help you find your way around each unit.

Did you know?

This parrot tells you where to find fun facts and information in our Did You Know boxes.

Case-study crab tells you where to find stories, poems and case studies.

Reflections give children something to think about by themselves.

There are lots of activities for children to enjoy. Afterwards discuss, ask questions about, and praise their work. **Activity**

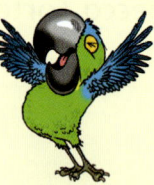 A single crab means children can do this activity by themselves.

Two crabs represents pair-work.

Three crabs means children should get into groups.

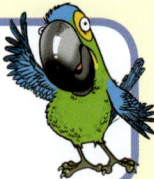 Four crabs means you can do this activity with the whole class.

Life Skills key steps are sometimes provided in boxes like this.

The bottom of each double page spread shows the theme and key life skills covered.

▶ **Key Life Skills: Communication**, Problem-solving, Self-awareness
▶ **Theme:** Self and Interpersonal Relationships

Refer to the Teacher's Guide for Level 2 for more information on how to teach HFLE: www.macmillan-caribbean.com

What are goals?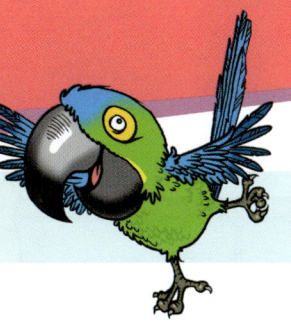

Goals are the things we aim at. They help us to plan for the future.

Some goals are for next week.
Some goals are for next year.
Some goals are for when you grow up.

Activity 2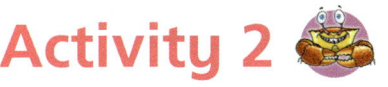

Write down:
1 One goal for tomorrow.
2 One goal for next week.
3 One goal for when you grow up.

Activity 3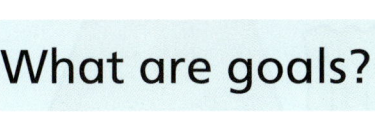

With your partner, talk about:
1 What you want to **DO** when you are an adult.
2 What you want to **BE** when you grow up.

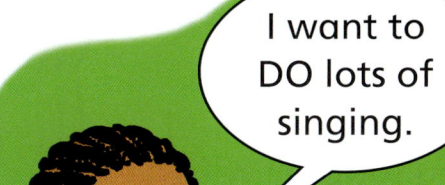

"I want to DO lots of singing."

"I want to BE a truck driver."

Goals help us to work hard.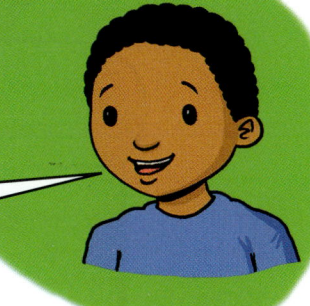

Goals help us to become the people we want to be.

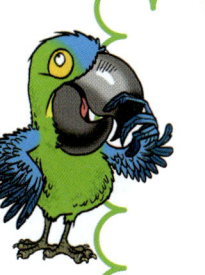

Reflection

I will think of three different jobs I might like to do when I grow up. Do these jobs fit with my likes and talents?

▶ Theme: Self and Interpersonal Relationships

SELF AND INTERPERSONAL RELATIONSHIPS

2 Making Decisions

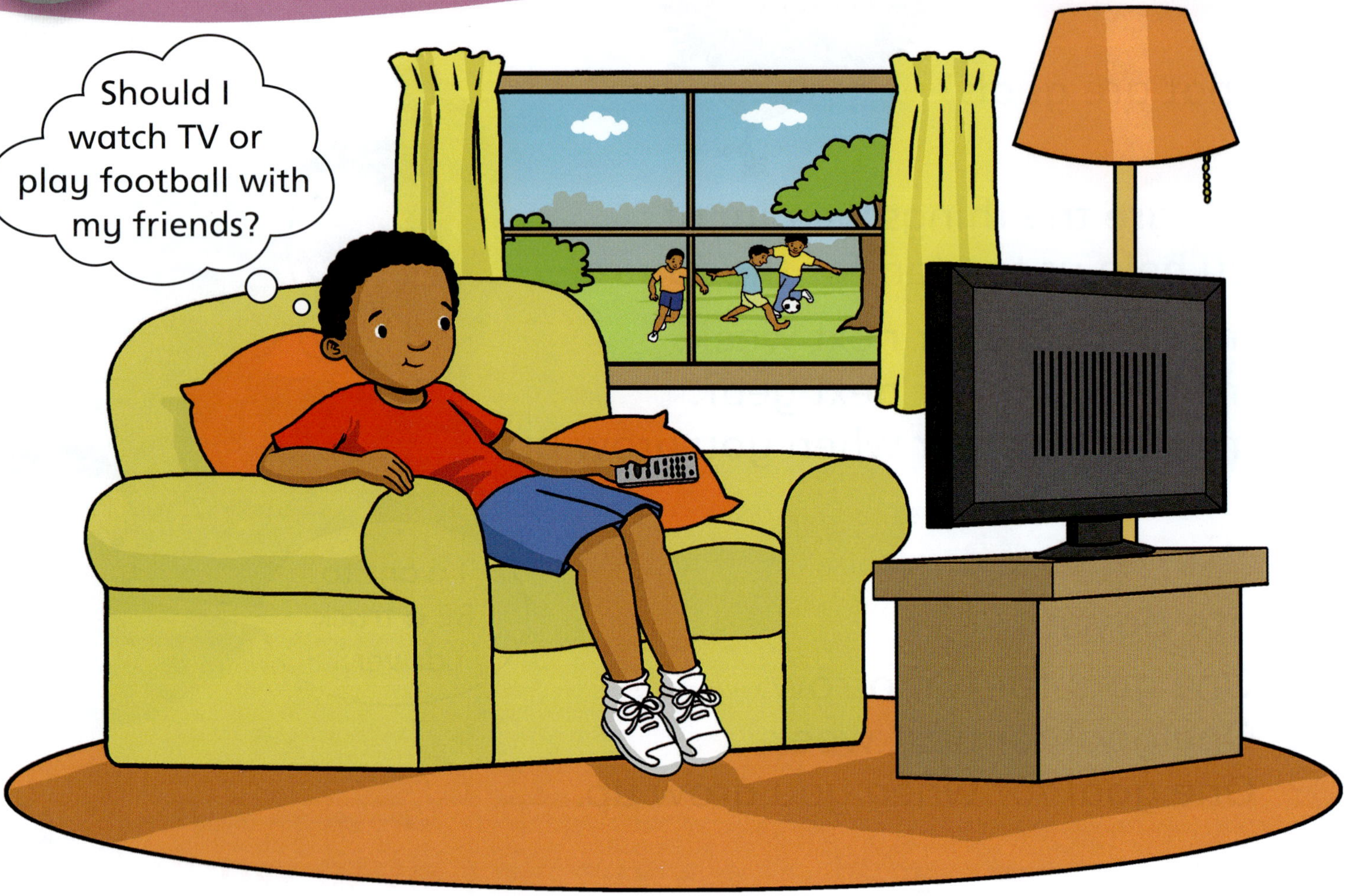

Should I watch TV or play football with my friends?

Activity 1

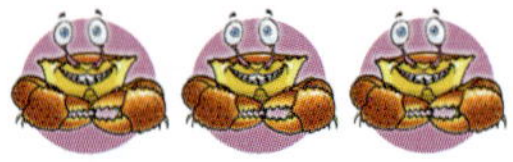

Look at the picture. Sean needs to make a decision. Talk with your group.

1. How can Sean decide what to do?
2. What options does he have?
3. What are the consequences of each option?
4. What do you think is the best decision and why?

Did you know?

Guessing is not smart, especially when you have an important decision to make.

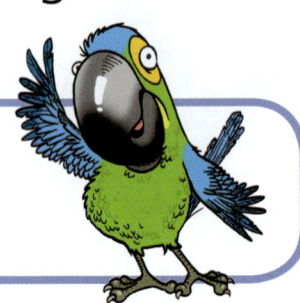

▶ Key Life Skills: **Decision-making,** Critical thinking, Self-awareness

Decision-making skills key steps

- What are the options?
- What are the consequences?
- Choose the best option.
- Act.
- Review the decision.

Activity 2

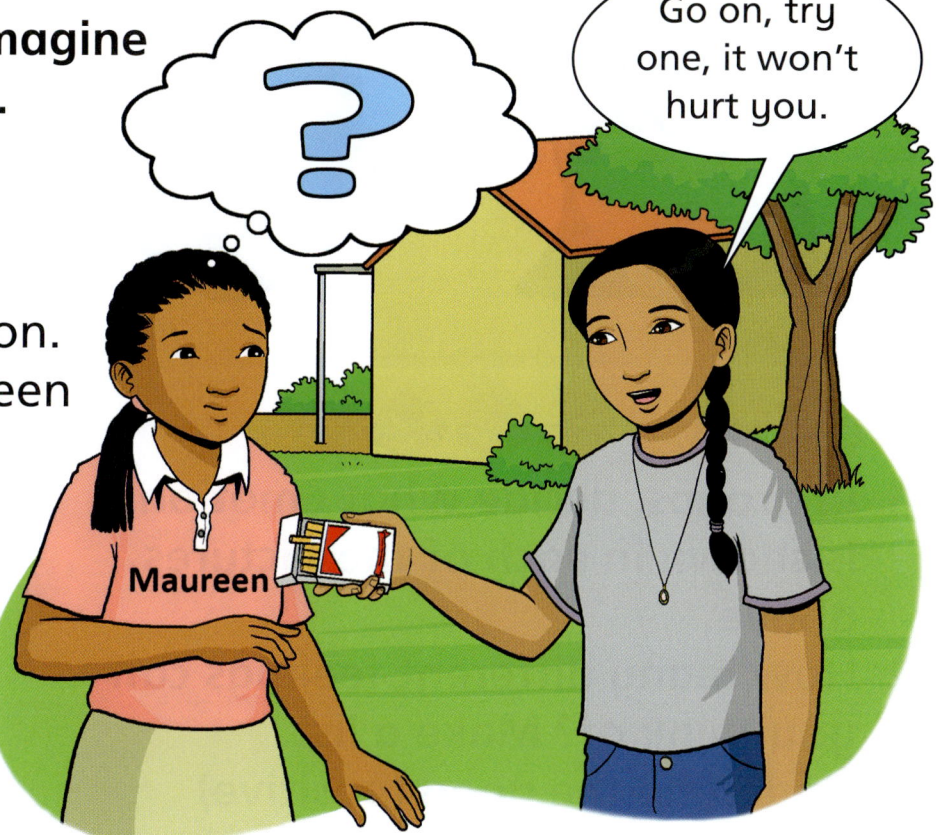

"Go on, try one, it won't hurt you."

Maureen

1 **With a partner, imagine you are Maureen.**
   - Write down the options and consequences.
   - Make the decision.
   - Role-play Maureen and her friend. What does Maureen say?
2 **How do you think Maureen feels about her decision?**

Share your ideas with the class.

Reflection

Do I watch too much TV? Do I arrive at school late? Can I make a decision to improve what I do?

▶ Theme: Self and Interpersonal Relationships

SELF AND INTERPERSONAL RELATIONSHIPS

Understanding Feelings

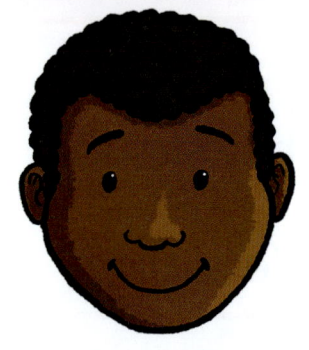 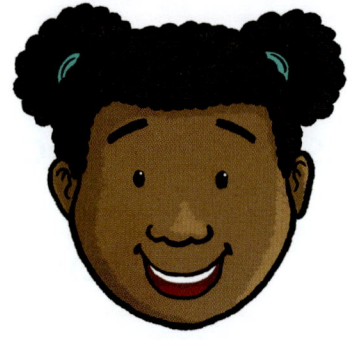 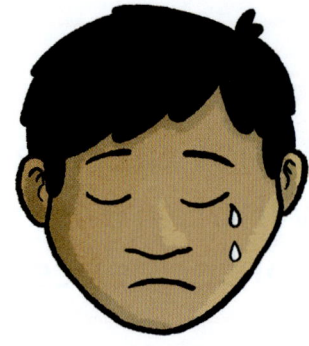

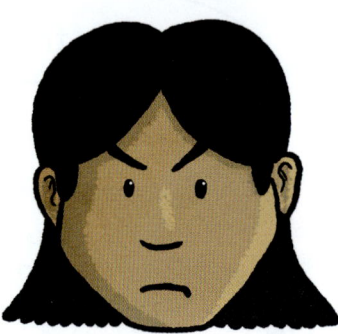 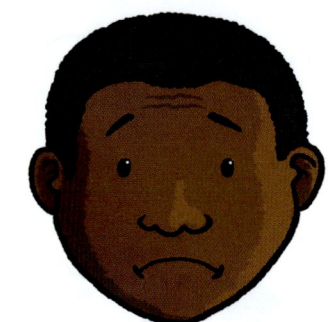 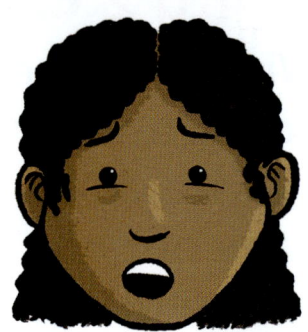

Activity 1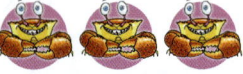

1. In groups, decide what emotion is shown in each of the pictures above.
2. How many different feelings can you think of? Make a list.
3. Underline the good (positive) feelings.
4. Circle the bad (negative) feelings.
5. Share your ideas with the class.

We all have different feelings or emotions. Some feel good, but others feel bad, uncomfortable or painful.

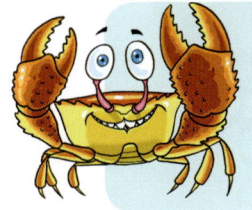

Feelings are caused by our experiences. Positive or good experiences cause happy feelings. Negative or bad experiences cause painful or sad feelings.

8 ▶ Key Life Skills: **Self-awareness,** Communication, Coping with emotions

Activity 2

1. What situations can make someone feel joyful, confident, hopeful or glad?
2. What situations can make someone feel anxious, angry, sad, lonely or afraid?

Match feelings to experiences

Our feelings cause us to behave in different ways. How do you behave when you feel happy? How do you behave when you feel sad or angry?

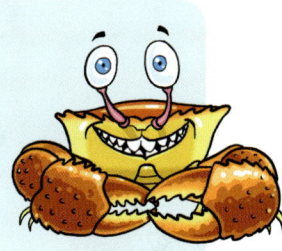

Activity 3

Choose a positive feeling and a negative feeling. For each, tell your partner how you feel and behave. Show facial expressions and body movements.

Sometimes when we feel bad we hurt other people or we dislike ourselves.

Activity 4

What makes you feel better when you have negative feelings? Share your ideas with a partner.

Reflection
How could I make a friend feel better?

▶ Theme: Self and Interpersonal Relationships

SELF AND INTERPERSONAL RELATIONSHIPS

4 Family Relationships

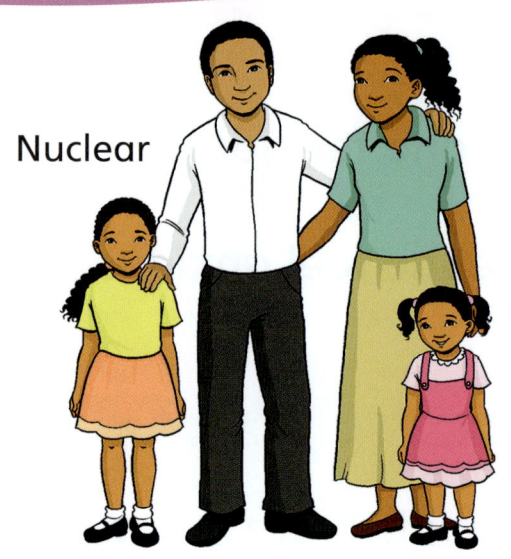

Nuclear

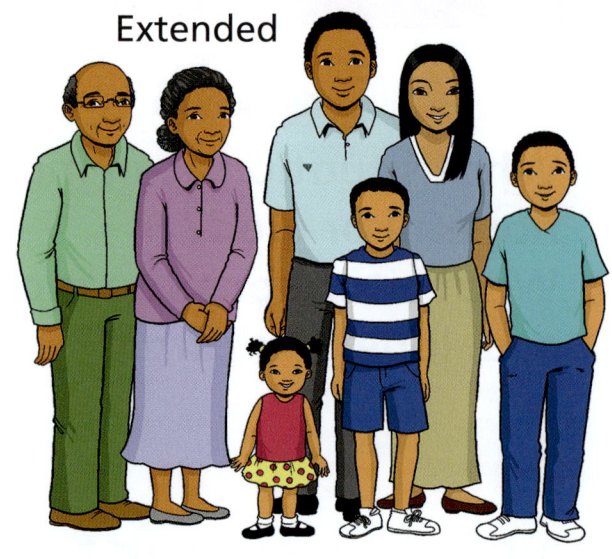

Extended

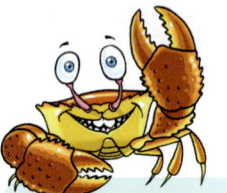

What is a family? What kind of family do you live in?

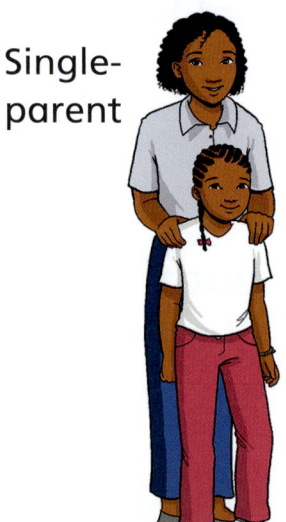

Single-parent

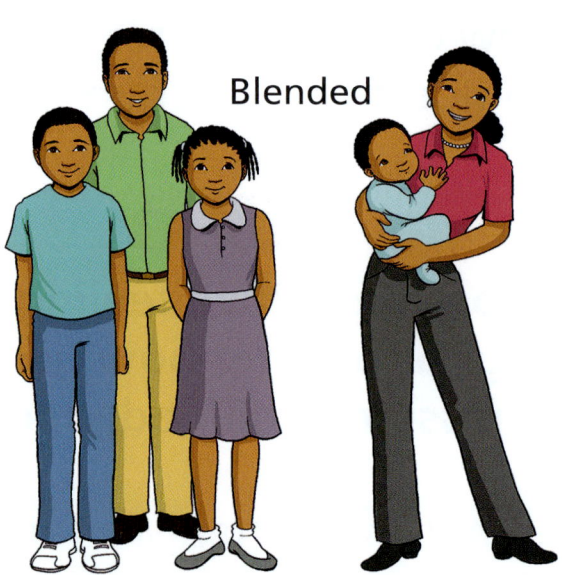

Blended

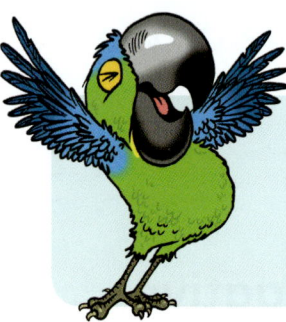

Usually some family members live together in the same household. Other family members may live elsewhere.

Activity 1

In small groups:
1. Talk about the members of your family.
2. Which family members live together in your household?
3. How many generations are there in your family?

▶ **Key Life Skills:** Interpersonal relations, Empathy, Self-awareness

Joe's family

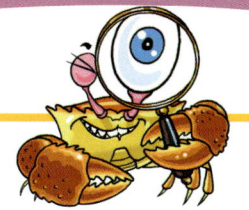

Joe is seven. He lives with his mother, grandmother and older sister Bella. His father often visits at weekends. Joe likes to spend time with his family. Sometimes they all go out together for a picnic or a walk to the beach. Sometimes Joe helps his grandmother to bake cakes and they talk. Joe and Bella often play football, or they draw pictures. Sometimes, in the evenings, Joe's mother reads to him. Best of all, Joe likes it when his father takes him to watch cricket. Joe feels a special bond with his father because they both like cricket.

Activity 2

1. What activities do all Joe's family do together?
2. How does Joe spend time with just his sister, his grandmother, his mother and his father?
3. How does the time they spend together help Joe's family to understand and like each other?
4. How does Joe feel about his father? Why does he feel this way?
5. How do your family spend time together?

Reflection

How do I feel about my family? How does spending time with my family help to build relationships?

▶ Theme: Self and Interpersonal Relationships

SELF AND INTERPERSONAL RELATIONSHIPS

5 Building Relationships

Most of us have people in our lives who we get along with well or who we particularly like. When we feel close to someone we share feelings with them and trust them. We feel safe and comfortable with them. We want to spend time with them.

Activity 1

Share with your partner the name of a person you feel close to. Explain how that makes you feel when you are with them and when you are away from them.

Did you know?

A **bond** is a tie. It can also mean a glue sticking things together. When we feel a special bond with someone we feel a connection to them.

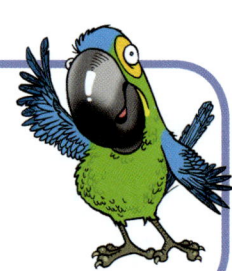

People may feel connected to each other for different reasons:

- They share the same personality, for example, Joe in Unit 4 is like his father.
- They like doing the same things, for example, watching cricket.
- They have had the same experiences.
- One person has been very kind to another.

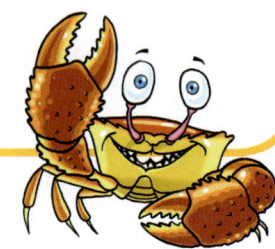

▶ Key Life Skills: **Empathy**, Communication, Interpersonal relations

Helping relationships to grow

Activity 2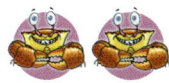

Think about the people you have relationships with, apart from your family. Do you have friends at school? Do you belong to any clubs or share activities with others? Share your ideas with your partner.

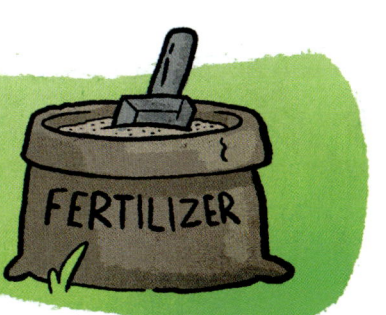

A relationship is like a plant – it grows well when we look after it.

We can help relationships to grow by looking after them:
- We can spend time together.
- We are kind to each other.
- We give each other support and help.
- We listen to each other and share.

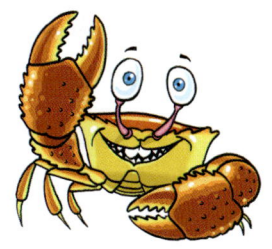

Activity 3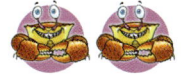

Role-play how you can help a friendship to grow. What can you say? What can you do?

Reflection

How can I help my relationships to grow?

▶ Theme: Self and Interpersonal Relationships

SELF AND INTERPERSONAL RELATIONSHIPS

6 Special Feelings

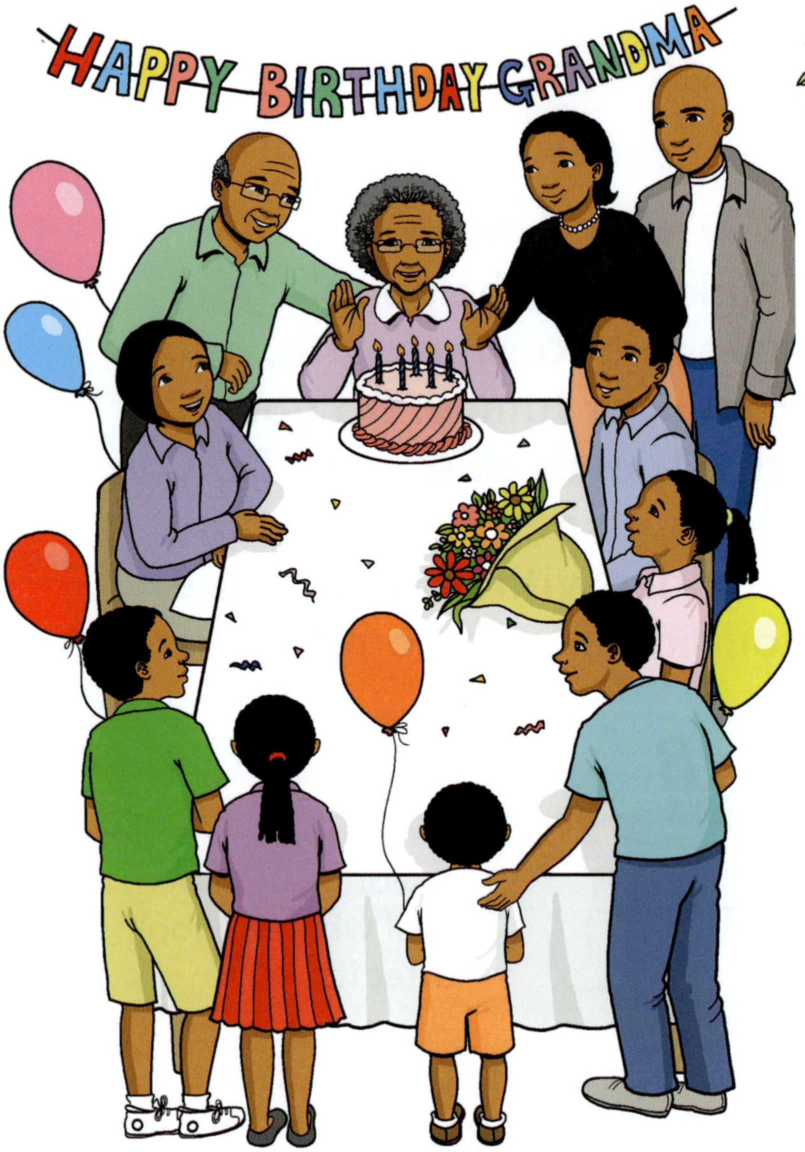

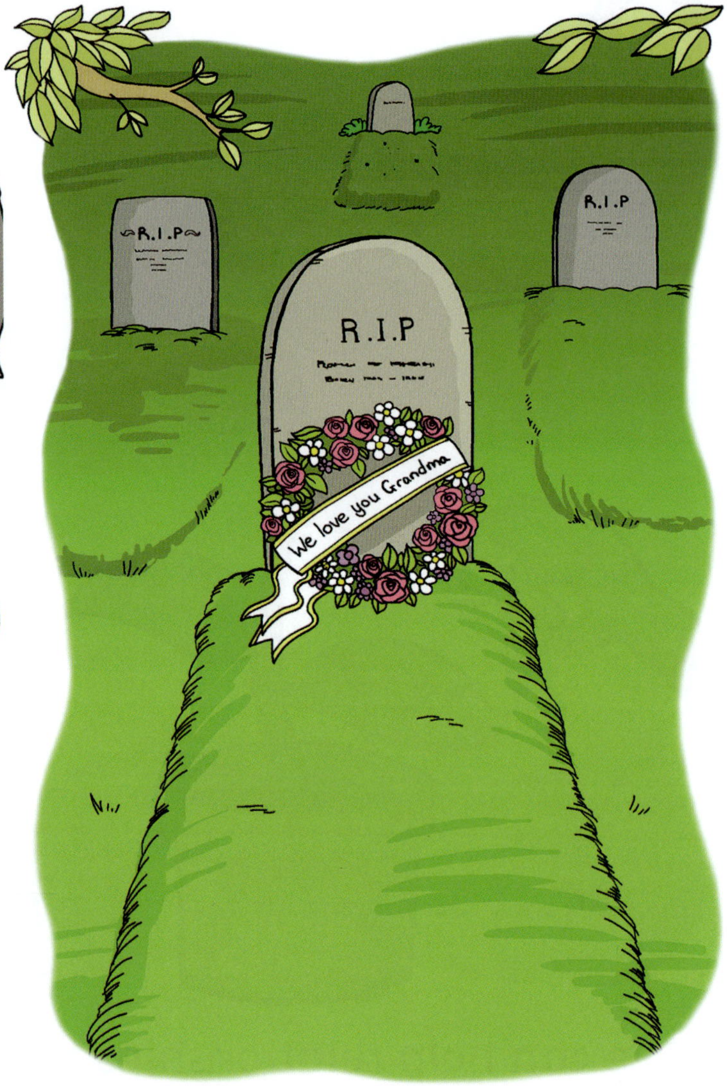

Activity 1

Get into groups and look at the two pictures.

1. What does the picture on the left show?
2. What feelings do people have at this occasion?
3. How do people express these feelings?
4. What has happened in the picture on the right?
5. How do people feel on this occasion?
6. How do people express these feelings?

14 ▶ Key Life Skills: **Communication,** Coping with emotions, Self-awareness

Activity 2
In groups, role-play Grandma's birthday party.

When do we feel sad?
- If we lose someone close to us, when they die.
- If we lose a family pet.
- If we lose a family member or good friend because they move away.
- If someone lets us down or we are disappointed.

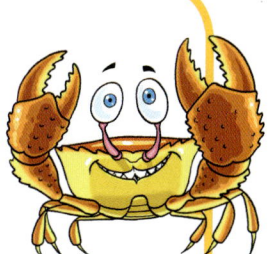

Activity 3
In groups, role-play visiting Grandma's grave or another situation where you feel sad.

Activity 4
With your partner, role-play helping someone who feels sad. Take it in turns to be the sad person and the helper.

Reflection
What makes me feel better if I am sad?
How can I help someone else to feel better?

▶ Theme: Self and Interpersonal Relationships

7 I Am Changing

SELF AND INTERPERSONAL RELATIONSHIPS

People and things do not stay the same. We are growing and changing.

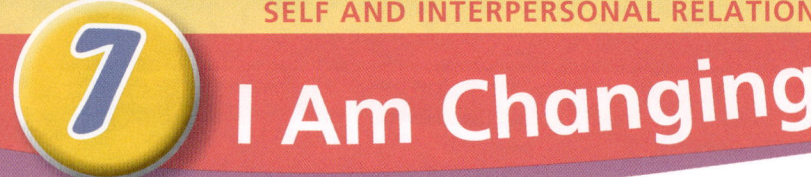

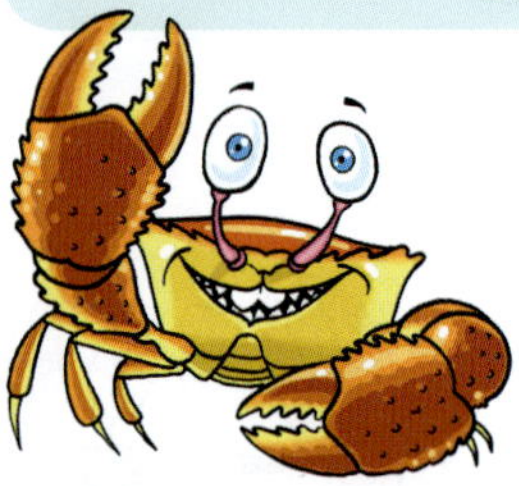

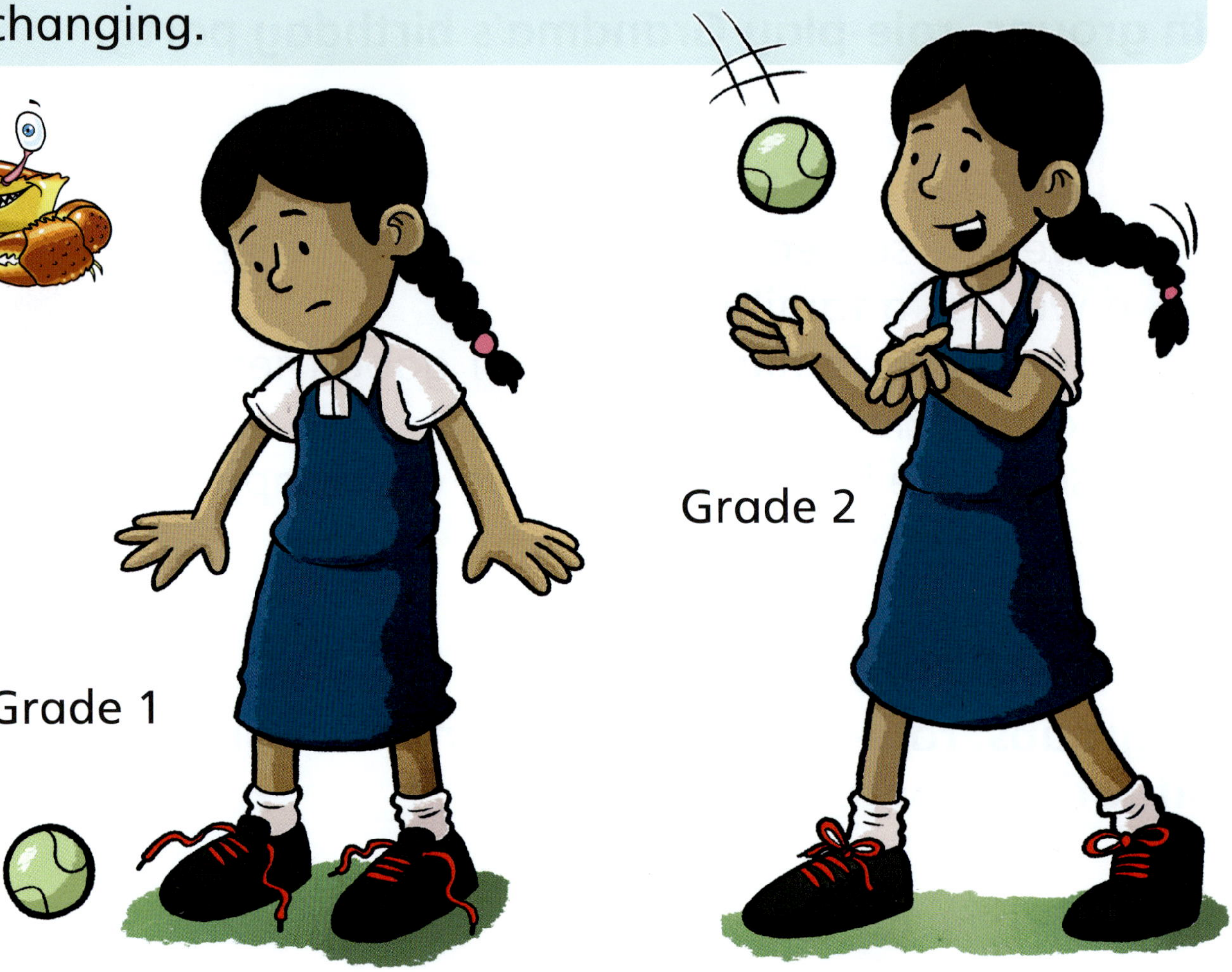

Grade 1

Grade 2

When Marcia started school, at the beginning of Grade 1, she was six. She could dress herself, say please and thank you (usually), read and write her name. She could not tie shoelaces, read stories, write sentences, or catch a ball. She didn't have any friends at school.

Now Marcia is in Grade 2. She is seven. She is taller and heavier than when she was six. She can read stories, write sentences and play ball. She can do lots of other things too. She has lots of friends in class now.

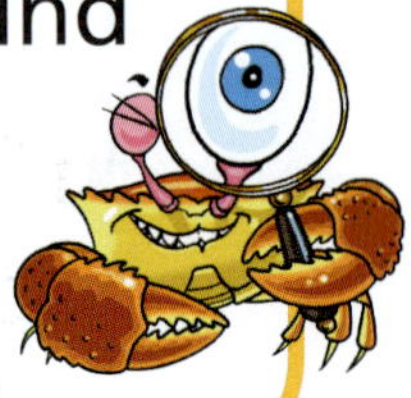

▶ Key Life Skills: **Self-awareness**, Communication, Decision-making

Activity 1

Discuss in groups:

1. What can Marcia do now that she couldn't do at the beginning of Grade 1?
2. What other things do you think Marcia might be able to do now?
3. What can you do now which you couldn't do at the beginning of Grade 1? How have you changed?

Some changes are good: when we learn new things or make new friends. Other changes can feel frightening, such as when we first start school. Marcia was worried about starting school, and about moving from Grade 1 to Grade 2.

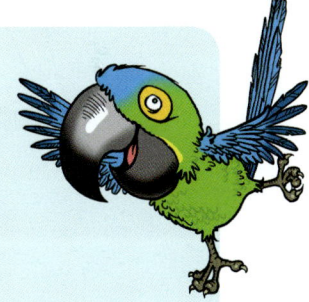

Activity 2

1. **Share one good change that has happened to you.**
2. **Share one change you have felt frightened or worried about.**

We all experience changes and we all change through our lives.

Reflection

What changes have happened to me in the last year? How do I feel about these changes?

▶ Theme: Self and Interpersonal Relationships

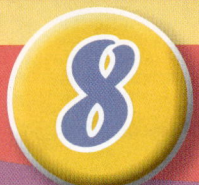

SELF AND INTERPERSONAL RELATIONSHIPS

8 Dealing with Changes

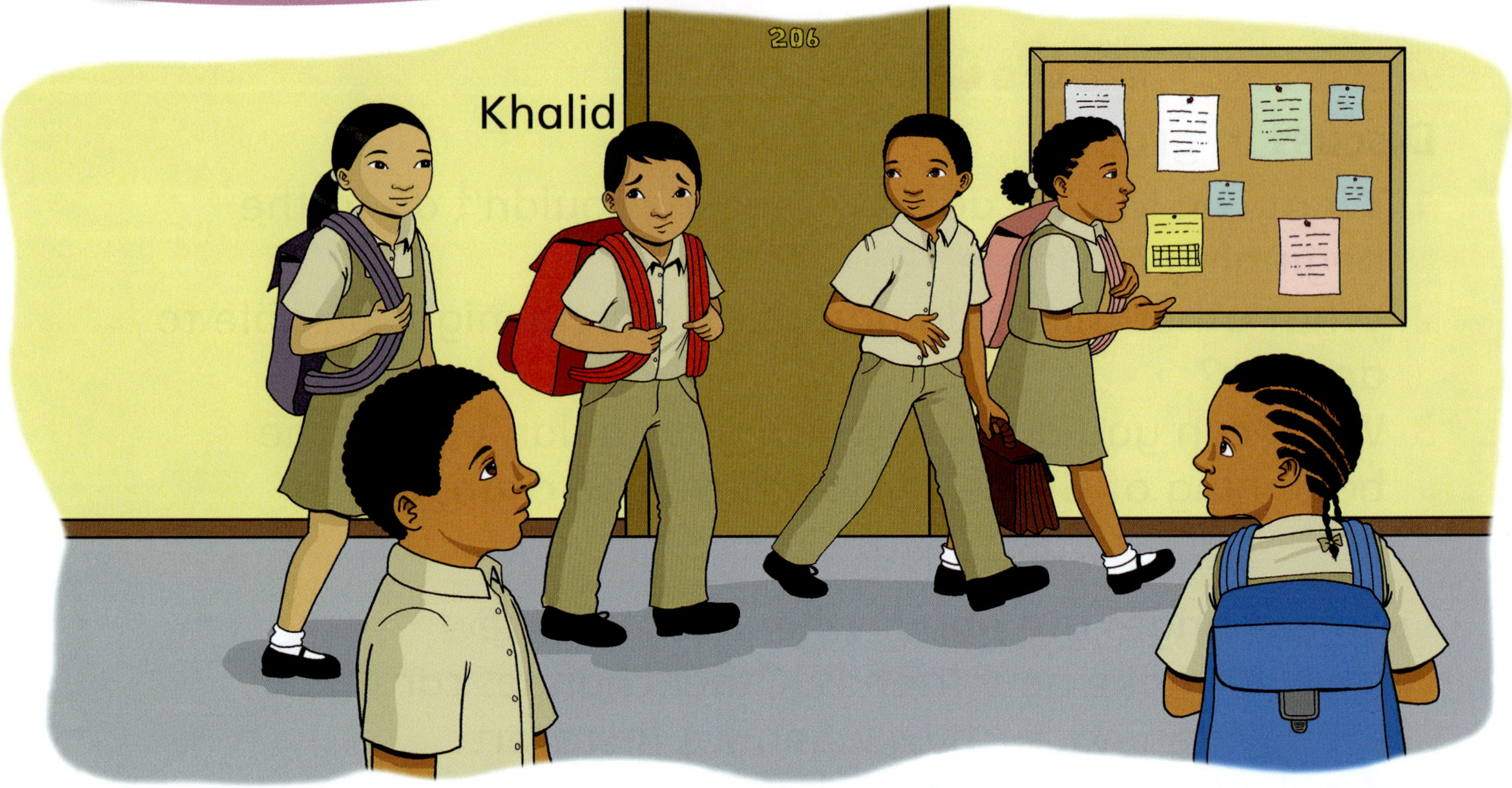

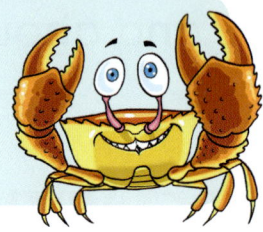

Sometimes things change. When Khalid's family moved from a village into the city he had to go to a new school. He did not know anyone.

Activity 1

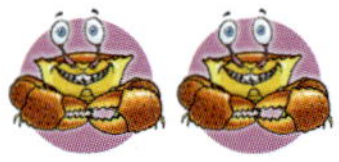

1 How do you think Khalid felt in the morning before he went to the new school?
2 How do you think Khalid felt when he arrived?
3 Who should Khalid speak to if he is worried or afraid?
4 How might he have felt by the time he went home that first day?
5 How can Khalid manage his feelings? How can he help himself to feel better?

Share your ideas with the class.

▶ Key Life Skills: **Self-management**, Communication, Critical thinking

Activity 2

In groups, role-play Khalid at break with his new classmates and the teacher.

- What does the teacher say?
- What do the classmates say?
- What does Khalid say?

Afterwards, talk about how each person felt and how they behaved.

Self-management skills key steps

- Name the feeling I am having.
- What causes it?
- How does it make me behave?
- What are the effects of my behaviour?

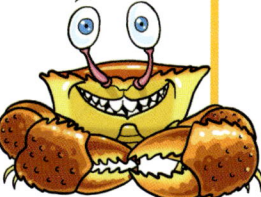

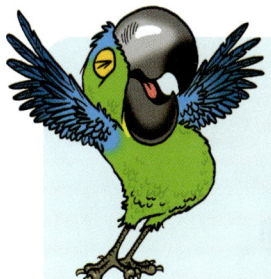

Sometimes there are sudden changes or problems. We may feel afraid or worried about what might happen to us. But we can learn to manage these changes and our own feelings.

Activity 3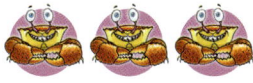

In your groups, think about the following changes. How would the child feel? What should they do? Where should they go for help?

1. Susie moves to a new neighbourhood and feels lonely.
2. Jack's father dies.
3. Heather's parents have to work overseas.
4. Melissa's mother is very ill.
5. Ray's uncle is drunk and tries to abuse him.

Reflection

Whom could I go to if I feel worried or afraid?

▸ Theme: Self and Interpersonal Relationships

SELF AND INTERPERSONAL RELATIONSHIPS

9 I Can Control Myself

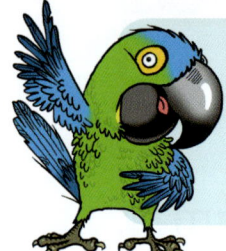

Paulette is seven. She is kind and friendly. She likes to play and laugh with her friends but sometimes she gets very angry.

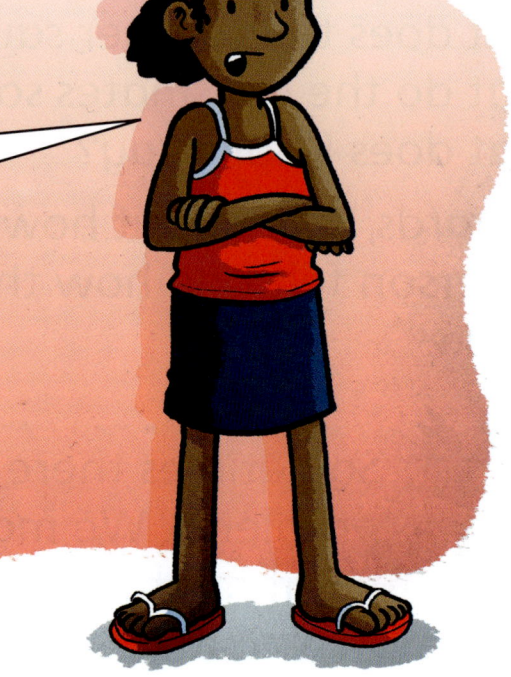

When I cannot do what I want I get very angry. I shout and stomp my feet. I don't like my angry self. What can I do about it?

Activity 1

Talk about the following questions in small groups, then carry out the role play.

1 What makes Paulette angry?
2 How does she behave?
3 How does Paulette feel about her angry self?
4 How do you think Paulette's behaviour affects others?

Now role-play Paulette getting angry at home or school when she cannot do something she wants to do.

We all get angry sometimes. It is OK to be angry, but it is never OK to hurt others, or ourselves, by actions or words.

▶ Key Life Skills: **Coping with emotions,** Interpersonal relations, Problem-solving

Ideas for dealing with anger safely:
- Walk away.
- Count to 10.
- Talk about how you feel.
- Punch the air or a cushion.
- Draw or write about your anger and screw up the paper.

Activity 2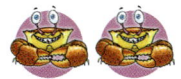
1. Suggest some ideas to help Paulette control her anger.
2. Role-play Paulette being told she cannot do something she wants to do and trying to control her anger.

Activity 3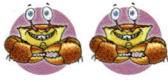
1. Share about a time when you got angry. What did you do and say?
2. Talk about what you could have done differently.

Apologies help
If you do get angry and hurt someone, then apologise afterwards. People will respect you and you will respect yourself again.

Activity 4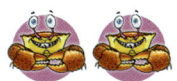
Role-play one person who got angry apologising to the other. Then swap over.

Reflection
What can I do to control my anger?

▶ Theme: Self and Interpersonal Relationships

SELF AND INTERPERSONAL RELATIONSHIPS

10 Communication

Communication means giving and receiving ideas and information. The most important ways we communicate are by speaking and listening.

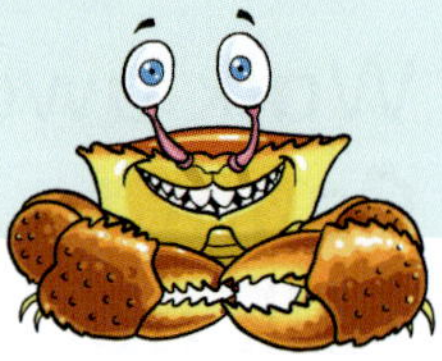

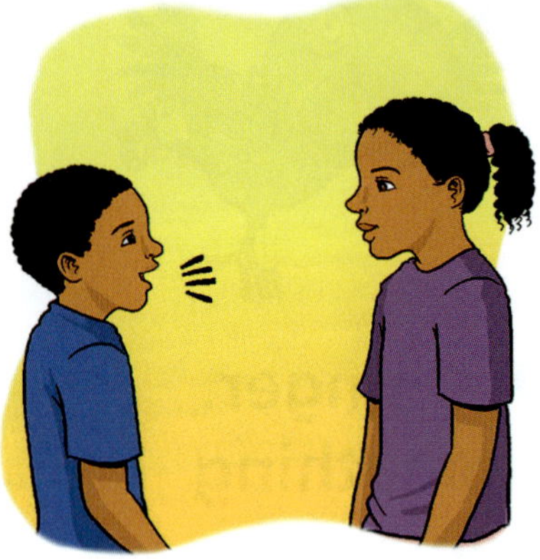

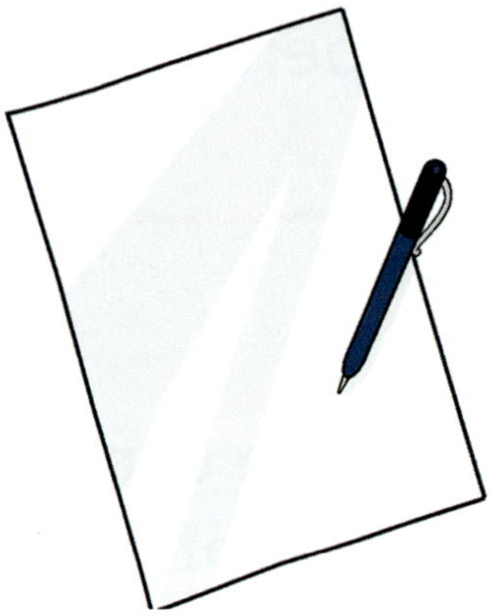

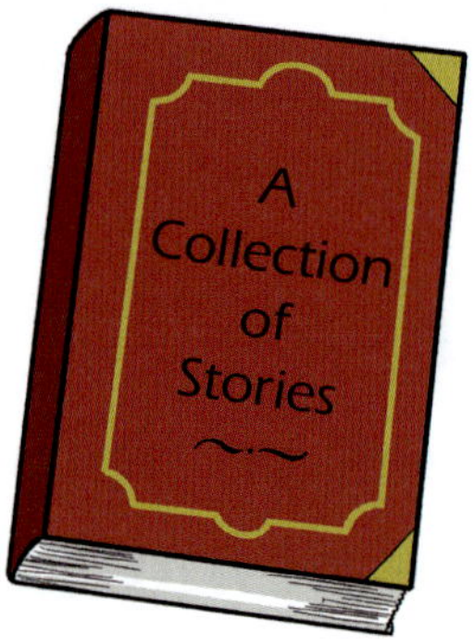

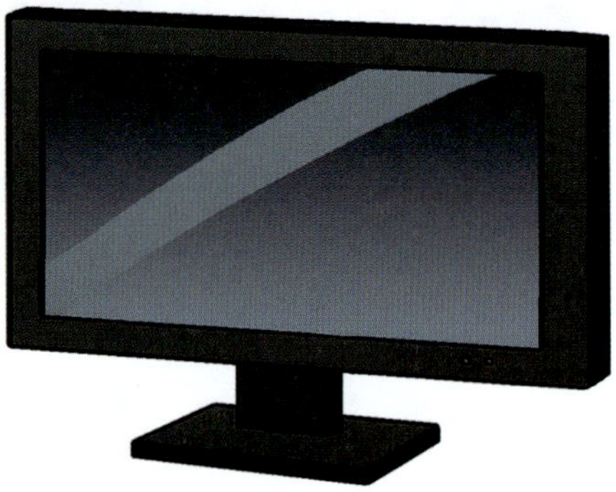

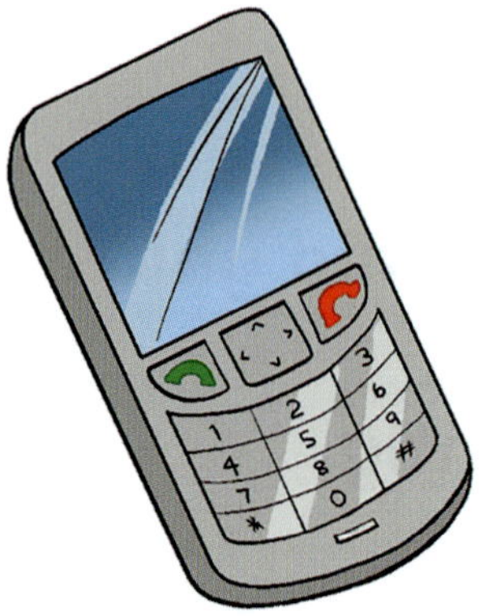

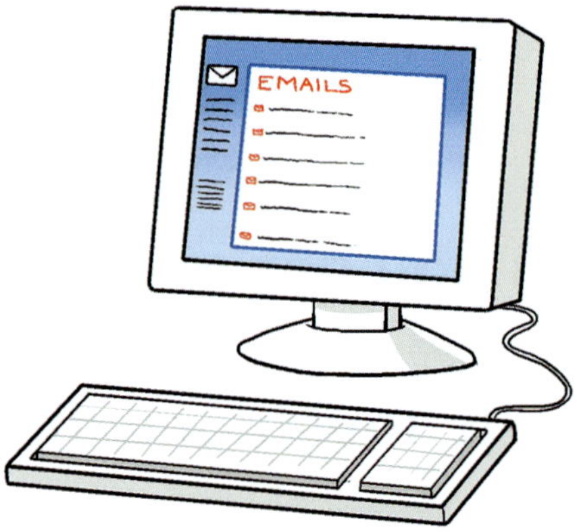

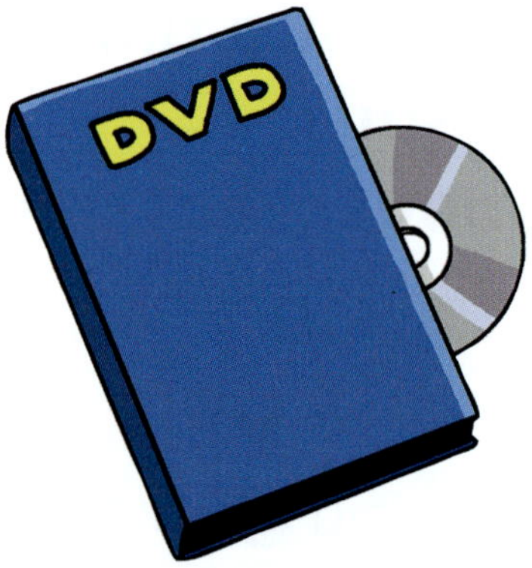

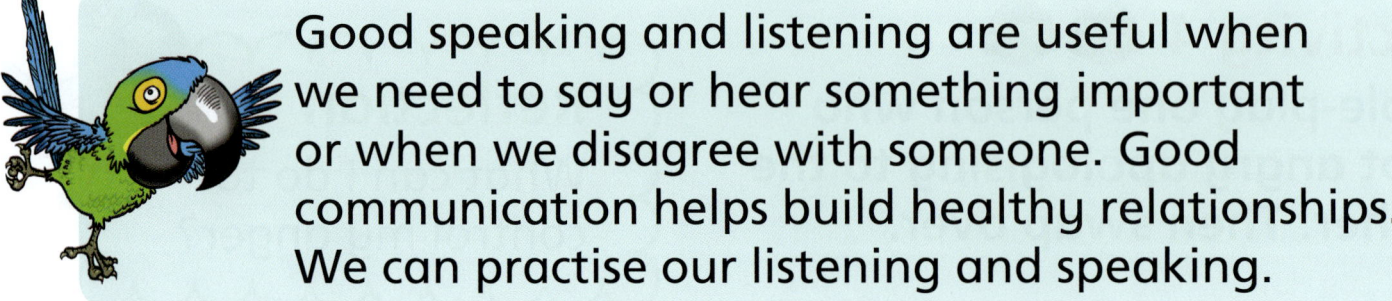

Activity 1

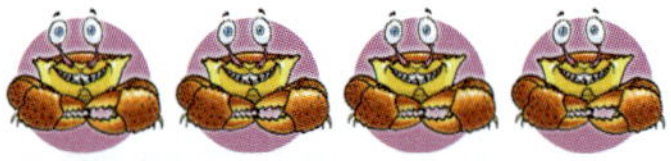

Look at the pictures. As a class:
1 Name the ways we communicate and the things we use.
2 Which of these ways do you use?

Good speaking and listening are useful when we need to say or hear something important or when we disagree with someone. Good communication helps build healthy relationships. We can practise our listening and speaking.

▶ Key Life Skills: **Communication,** Problem-solving, Decision-making

Listening skills key steps

- Keep eye contact.
- Listen carefully to the speaker's words.
- Watch the speaker's body language.
- Use your body: smile, nod, and so on.

Speaking skills key steps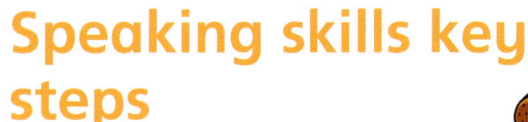

- Face the person and make eye contact.
- Wait for the other person to stop speaking before you speak.
- Speak clearly, not too fast.
- Watch the listener and their responses.

Activity 2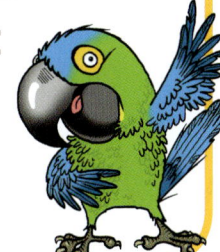

Practise your speaking and listening skills. Your teacher will give you something to talk about.

1. Take it in turns to be the speaker and the listener.
2. After each turn say what your partner did well.

Activity 3

Jason and Darren disagree. Jason wants to play football. Darren wants to play chase.

Role-play the conversation between Jason and Darren.

> ## Reflection
> How can I improve my listening and speaking skills?

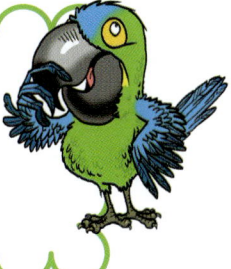

Theme: Self and Interpersonal Relationships

SELF AND INTERPERSONAL RELATIONSHIPS

11 Drugs

Drugs can be helpful or harmful. Medicines such as aspirin are helpful when we are ill. Drugs such as cigarettes, alcohol, cocaine, marijuana and heroin can harm our bodies, our minds and our health.

Some drugs are **legal** (allowed), such as medicines, cigarettes and alcohol.

Some drugs are **illegal** (against the law), such as cocaine, heroin and marijuana.

Did you know?

Cigarettes cause illnesses of the lungs and mouth: bronchitis, lung and mouth cancers. They affect people who smoke and also those who live with them.

If someone offers you drugs you should:

- Say 'No'.
- Use refusal skills.
- Tell someone you trust.
- Go to a safe place.

Margaret's story

Margaret is in her twenties. She has been drinking alcohol since she was 13. Alcohol affects her brain. It makes her clumsy so she can't walk straight. It affects her judgement so she doesn't know when she's in danger and takes risks. It affects her memory. Alcohol can cause cancers, liver and kidney disease.

▶ Key Life Skills: **Refusal skills,** Decision-making, Healthy self-management

Activity 1

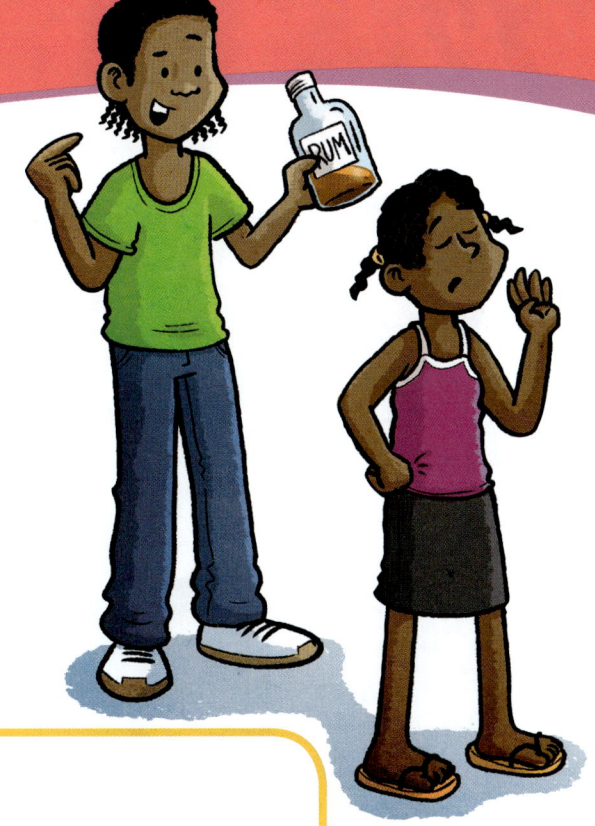

Answer the following questions in groups:
1. Name two harmful drugs
2. Name two illegal drugs.
3. Name two legal drugs.
4. How do cigarettes harm us?
5. What are some effects of alcohol?

Refusal skills key steps

- Say 'No'.
- Use a strong clear voice and keep eye contact.
- Do not smile.
- Repeat 'No' as often as necessary.
- If necessary, walk away.

Activity 2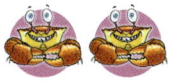

Role-play a situation where one of you offers the other one a cigarette. Use refusal skills. Swap over so both of you can practise your refusal skills.

Activity 3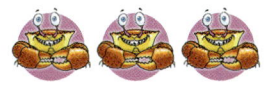

In groups of four, try to persuade one person to try alcohol. That person practises using refusal skills. Take turns.

Reflection

Is it harder to refuse a group of people than just one other person? Why?

▶ Theme: Self and Interpersonal Relationships

SELF AND INTERPERSONAL RELATIONSHIPS

12 Beautiful People

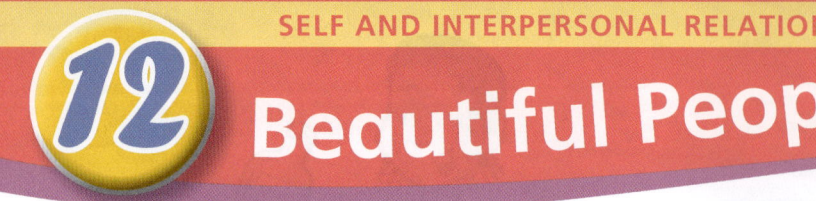

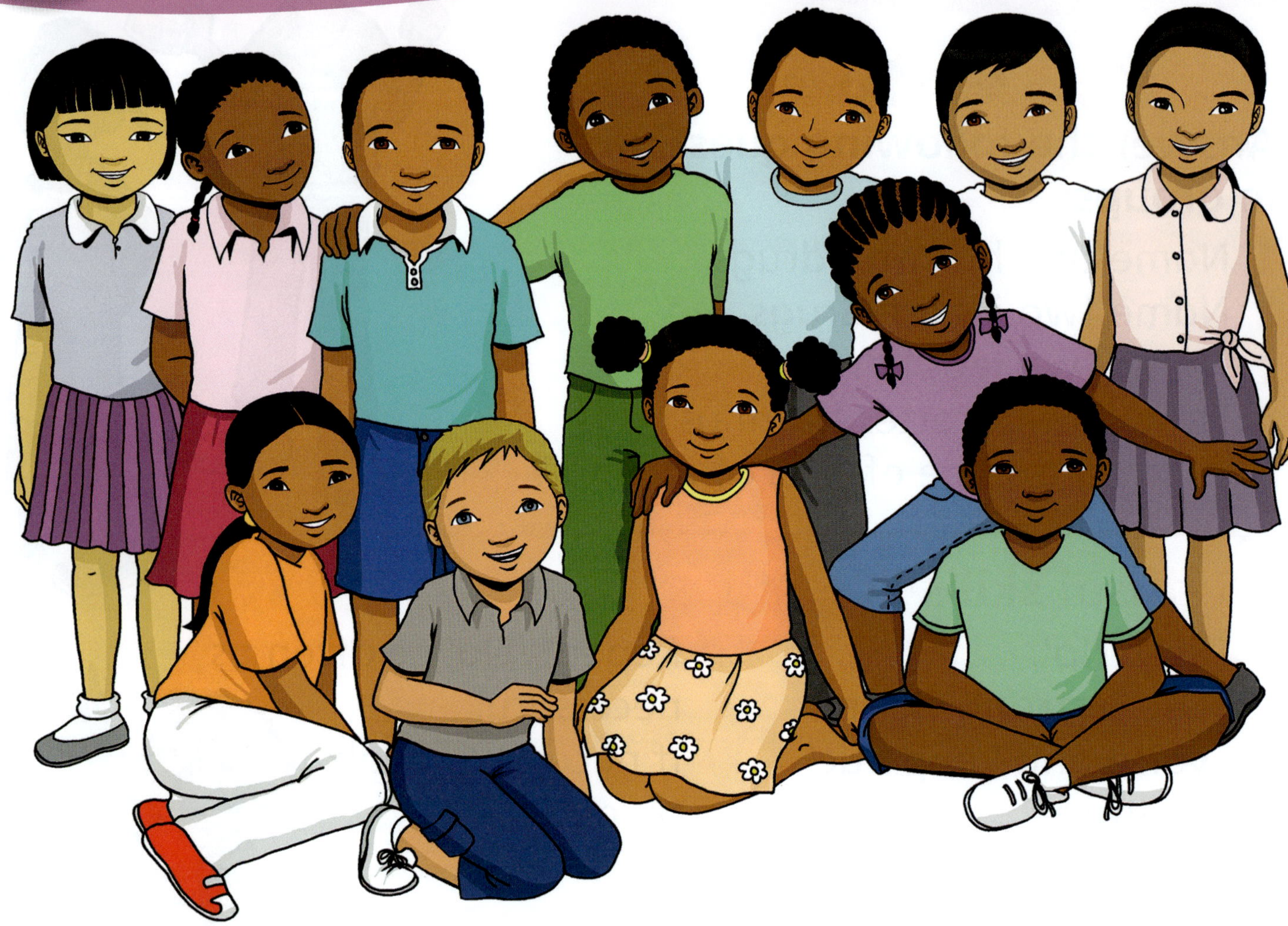

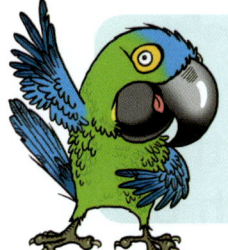

The children in the picture are all friends. They belong to different ethnic groups. Some are girls and some are boys.

Activity 1

In small groups, answer the questions:
1 How many different ethnic groups are in the picture?
2 How many boys and how many girls are there?
3 Which ethnic group do you come from?
4 Can you see children from your ethnic group in the picture?

▶ Key Life Skills: **Advocacy**, Creative thinking, Self-awareness

People of different ethnic groups have different cultures. Sometimes we eat different foods, wear different clothes and do different things. We have different religions and beliefs.

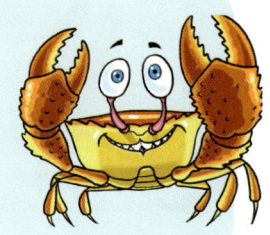

Activity 2

Role-play a scene from a celebration or festival which some children in your group celebrate.

Our rights

We are all equal. We have the same rights to:
- a name
- a home
- love and care.
- a family
- food and water

We need to get along with each other to make the world a better place.

Activity 3

Talk about why these rights are important in a class discussion.

Reflection

How can I stand up for other children's rights?

Theme: Self and Interpersonal Relationships

SEXUALITY AND SEXUAL HEALTH

1 Growing Up

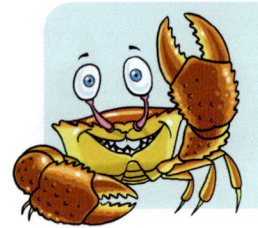 We all grow and change as we get older. We grow on the outside, and on the inside. We grow at different rates and different times.

Did you know?
It takes about 21 years for human beings to grow fully and become adult.

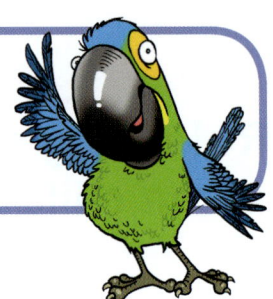

Activity 1

In groups, list five ways in which your bodies have changed since you were a baby.

Caring for our bodies

We need to look after our body parts such as hands, feet, faces, legs and trunk. We also need to look after our private body parts. We use these parts for going to the toilet and later, when we are adults, for making babies. We keep our private parts covered. We need to look after them and keep them clean.

Reflection
How can I look after my body better?

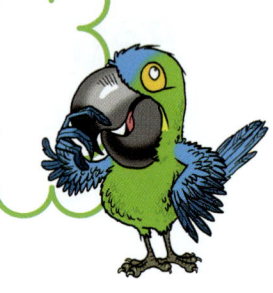

▶ Key Life Skills: **Critical thinking,** Communication, Self-awareness

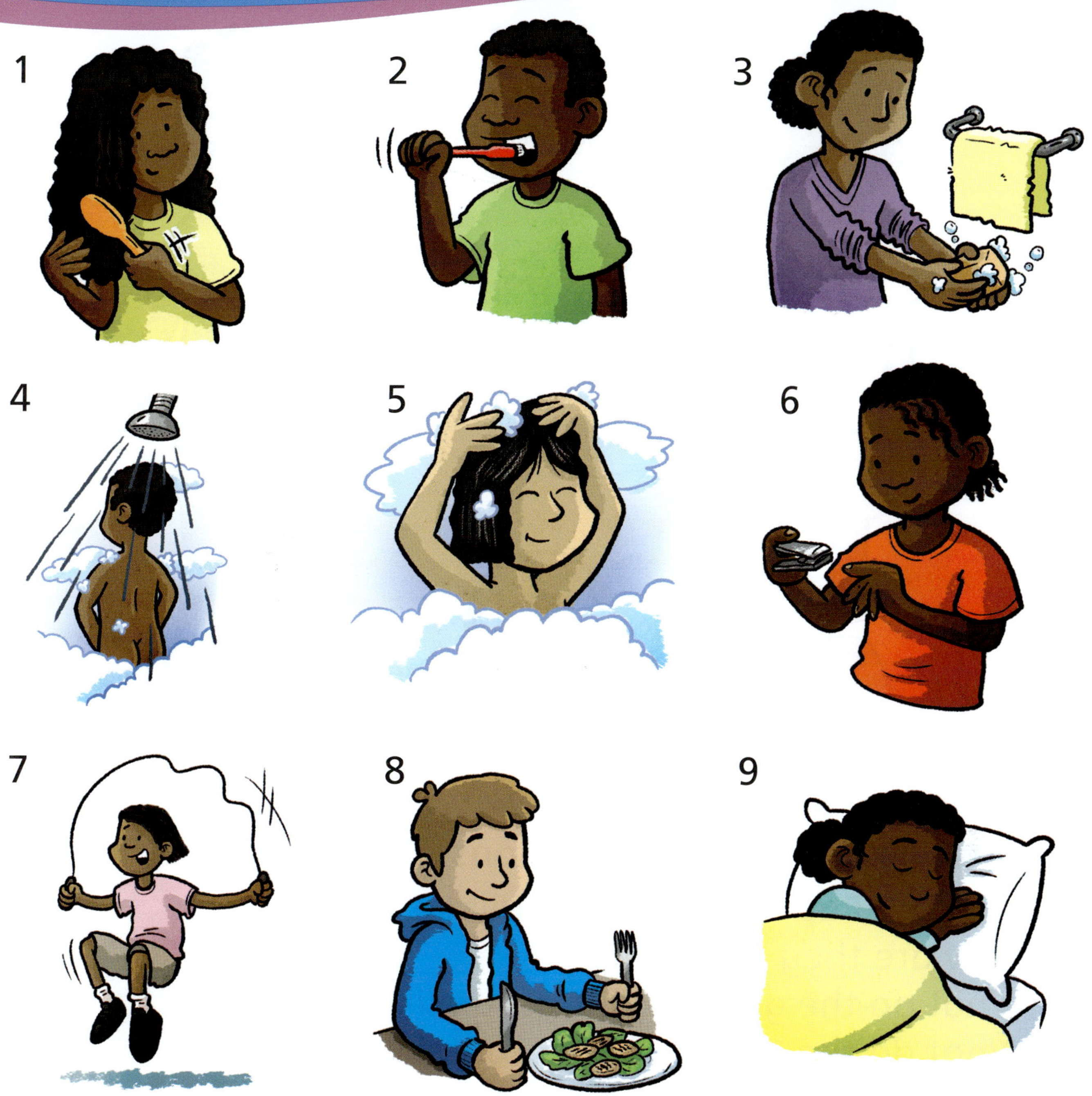

Activity 2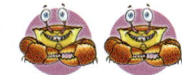

How do you care for your bodies? Look at the pictures.
1 What is happening in each picture?
2 Talk about when you do these things.
3 Practise washing your hands properly. Your teacher will show you how.

▶ Theme: Sexuality and Sexual Health

SEXUALITY AND SEXUAL HEALTH

2 Alike but Different

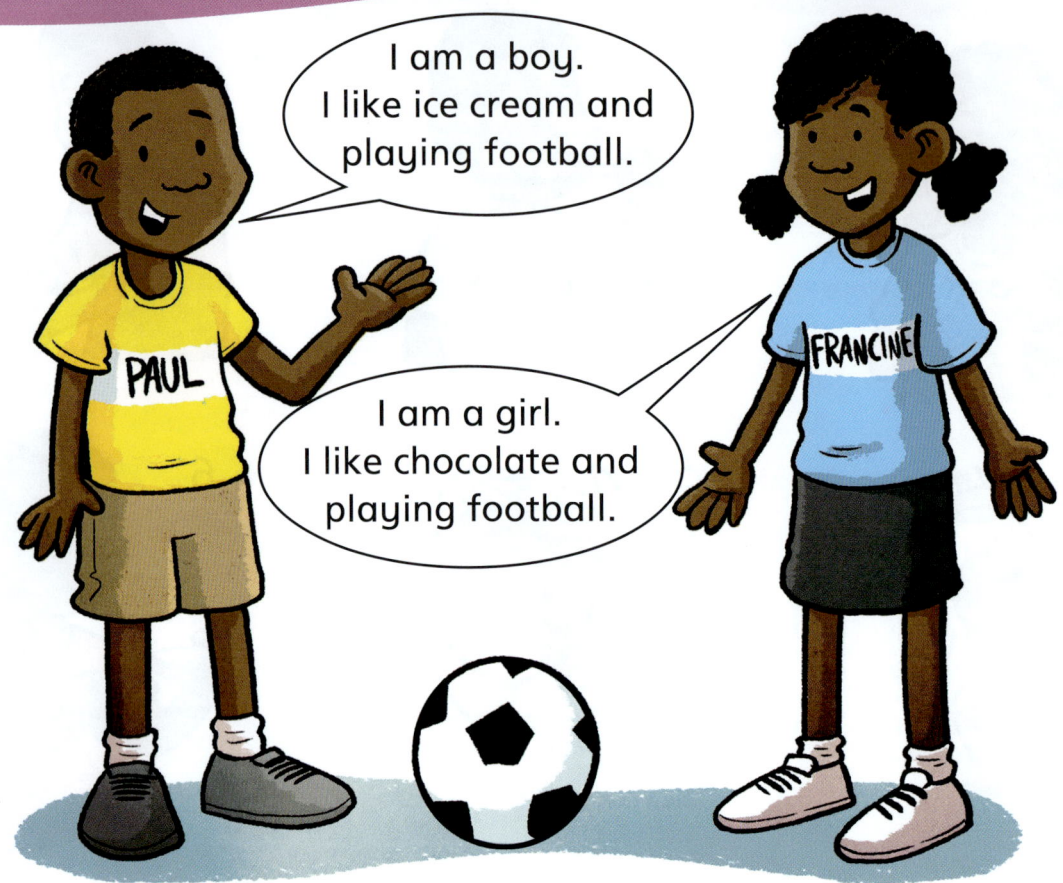

Activity 1

In groups, answer the questions.
1. How are Paul and Francine alike?
2. How are they different?
3. What do the girls in your group like to eat?
4. What do the boys in your group like to eat?
5. What do the girls and boys in your group like to do?

Did you know?

Our **sex** means whether we are male or female. Our **genders** (boys and men or girls and women) are the behaviours and dress that people expect from the different sexes.

Key Life Skills: **Critical thinking,** Communication, Self-awareness

Activity 2

With your partner, talk about the tasks (chores) which are done at home.

1 Which tasks do females (women and girls) do?
2 Which tasks do males (men and boys) do?
3 Can girls and boys do the same tasks? Why? Why not?

Share your ideas with the class.

> Our families, our communities and media like TV and radio, give us messages about the kinds of things we should do and how we should look as boys and girls. This starts when we are very young but carries on all our lives. But we do not always have to follow these messages.

Activity 3

As a class:

1 List some activities at school that both girls and boys can do.
2 List some activities which are reserved for either boys or girls.
3 Talk about: Is this fair? Why? Why not?

Reflection

I will think about activities I have in common with someone of the other gender. How do I feel about these activities?

▶ Theme: Sexuality and Sexual Health

SEXUALITY AND SEXUAL HEALTH

Good Touch, Bad Touch

Some touches feel good. Other touches feel bad.

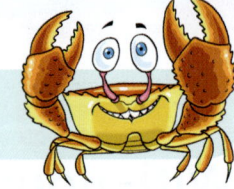

Did you know?

It is **not** OK for someone to touch your private parts even if:
- they are a member of your family
- they offer to pay for something or buy you something.

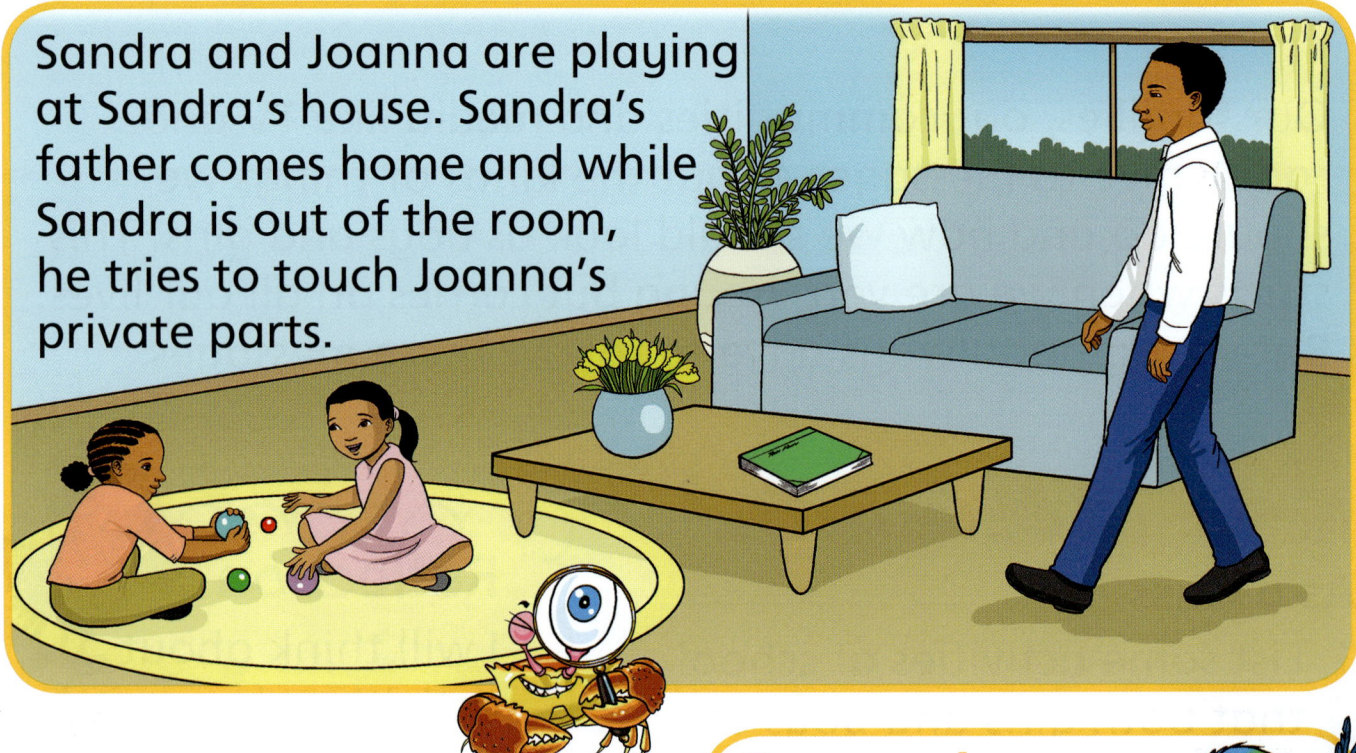

Sandra and Joanna are playing at Sandra's house. Sandra's father comes home and while Sandra is out of the room, he tries to touch Joanna's private parts.

Activity 1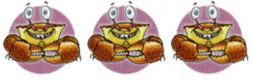

In groups, talk about:
1 What kind of touch is this?
2 Why is this risky for Joanna?
3 What should she do?

Remember: No! Go! Tell!

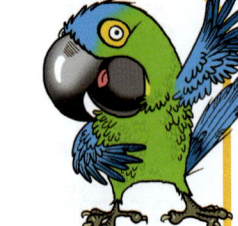

- Say **No!**
- **Go** away fast.
- **Tell** an adult you trust. If they do not believe you, tell someone else.

▶ Key Life Skills: **Assertiveness**, Decision-making, Refusal skills

Here are some more stories.

1. Ben and Simon are at the park. A man asks them to touch his private parts.
2. Louise is at the doctor's because she has a pain in her bottom. The doctor looks at her bottom and touches it.
3. Susannah is at home with a friend. Her brother asks them to play a game of taking off their clothes.
4. Nelson is on the computer. Someone asks him to upload a picture of himself naked.
5. John has trouble peeing into the toilet so his father shows him how to hold his penis to get a better aim.

Activity 2

With your partner, read the stories above.

1. Decide which ones are risky for the children involved and which ones are OK.
2. For the ones which are risky, decide what each child should do.
3. Choose one risky story and role-play saying 'No'.

Reflection

How could I be a friend to these children?

Activity 3

1. Share some good touches you give or receive.
2. Choose one kind of bad touch.
3. Talk about what you should do if you receive this bad touch.
4. Take turns to practise saying 'No' to a bad touch.

▶ Theme: Sexuality and Sexual Health

SEXUALITY AND SEXUAL HEALTH

4 HIV Prevention

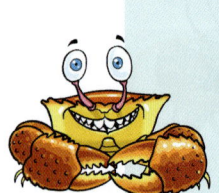

HIV is a kind of germ. It is a virus. It attacks our immune system, which protects us from disease. HIV can be treated but not cured. People with HIV are not able to fight the germs that cause diseases. When people with HIV become very ill with many diseases then they have AIDS.

People can have HIV for many years without knowing. During this time they can pass it on to others.

Did you know?

HIV is Human Immuno-deficiency Virus.
AIDS is Acquired Immuno-deficiency Disease Syndrome.

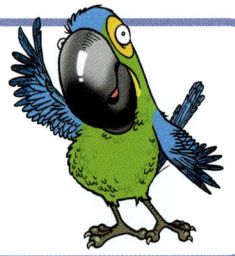

Activity 1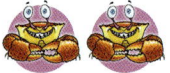

Read the text above.
1. What is HIV?
2. What part of the body does it affect?
3. Can HIV be treated?
4. Can HIV be cured?

HIV can be spread if infected blood enters someone else's body. So if there is an accident with blood, tell an adult immediately.

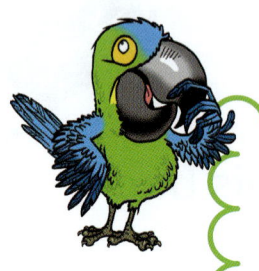

Reflection
What must I do to avoid getting HIV?

▸ Key Life Skills: **Creative thinking**, Communication, Decision-making

HIV is spread:

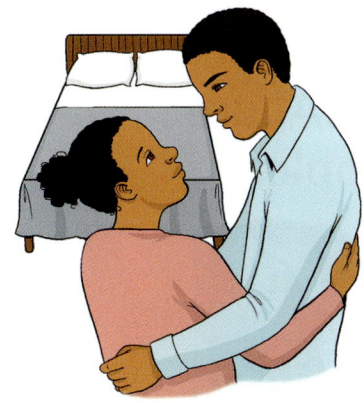
When someone has sex with a person who has HIV.

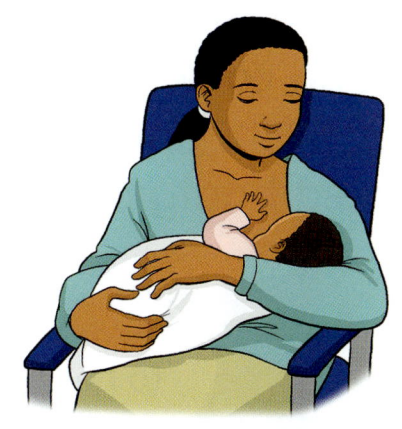
A mother with HIV can pass it to her baby.

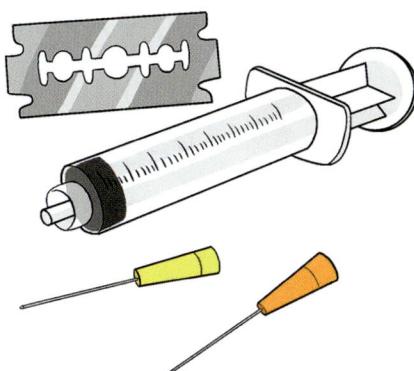
Through blood on unsterilised needles, syringes, razors and other instruments.

HIV is not spread by:

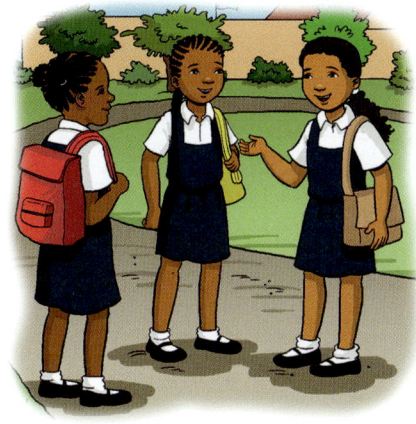
Being friends with someone.

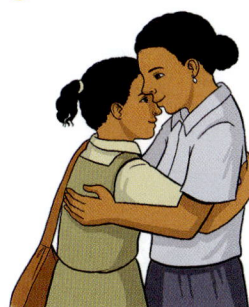
Hugging or shaking hands.

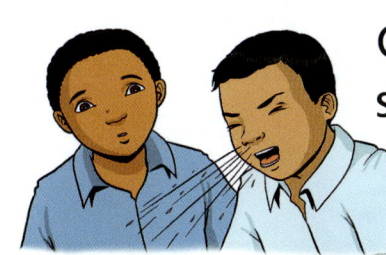
Coughs or sneezes.

Sharing cups, plates, knives and forks or food.

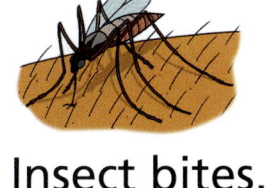
Insect bites.

HIV is not spread in saliva, tears, urine or faeces.

Activity 2

1. **Role-play what to do after a playground accident.**
2. **Make up a song or poem to tell other children how HIV is spread and not spread.**

▶ Theme: Sexuality and Sexual Health

SEXUALITY AND SEXUAL HEALTH

5 Caring for People with HIV and AIDS

We are all different and special individuals. We should respect and care for each other. People living with HIV and AIDS (PLWHA) are sometimes treated badly by other people.

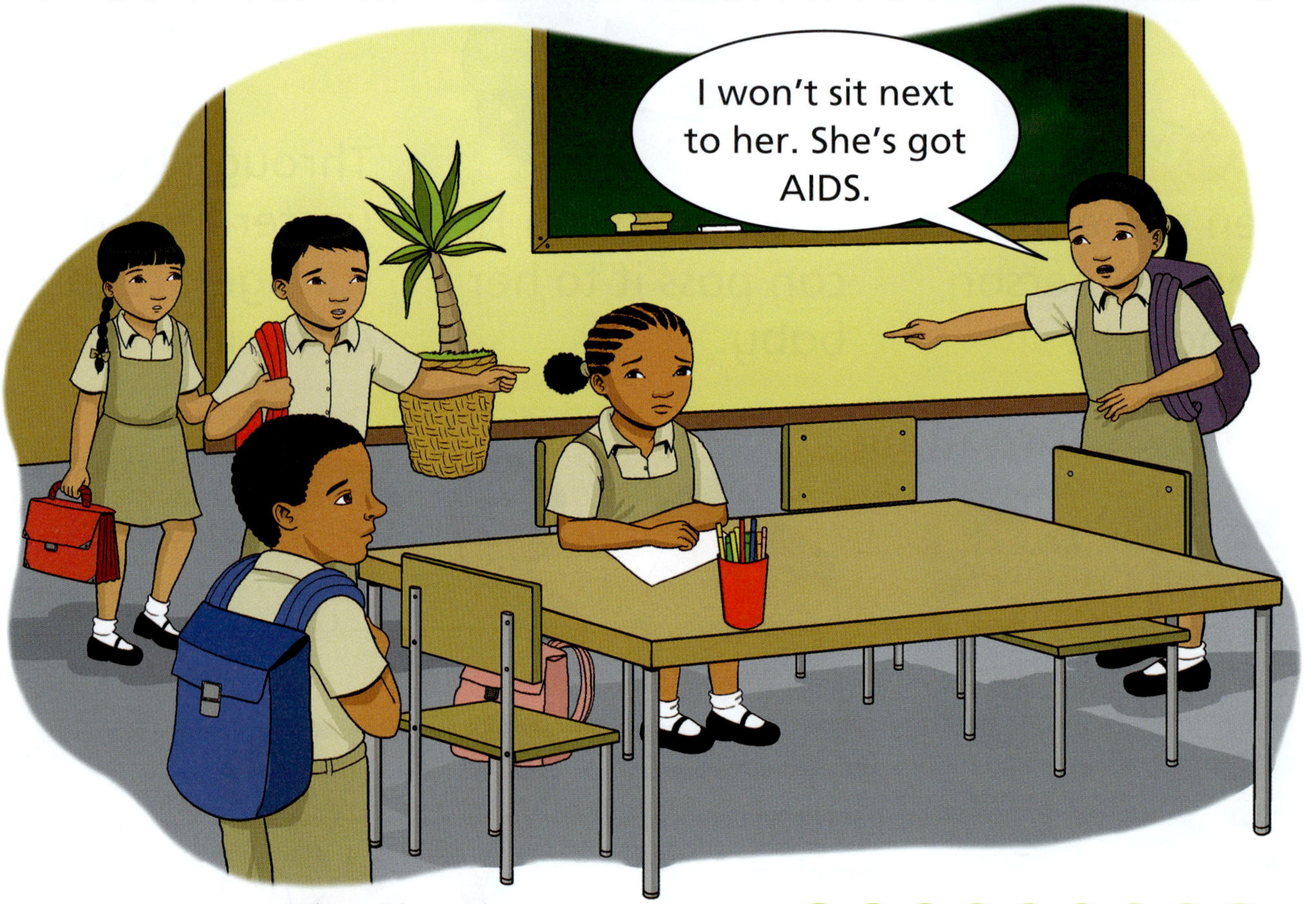

I won't sit next to her. She's got AIDS.

Activity 1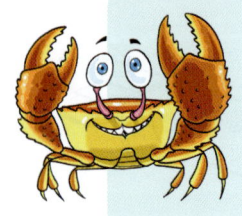

In groups, look at the picture.
1. Why do you think the other children won't sit with Saffron?
2. How are they behaving?
3. How does Saffron feel?
4. What can the teacher do to help the situation?

Reflection
Am I always kind to others? How can I improve my care of other people?

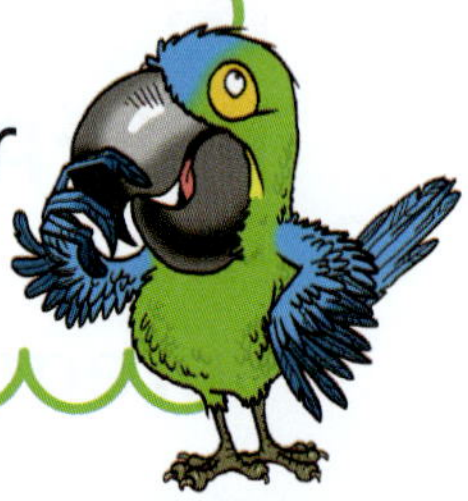

▶ Key Life Skills: **Empathy**, Advocacy, Coping with emotions

Activity 2

In groups, role-play the situation shown in the picture. Show what happens after the picture to make a good ending for Saffron.

People who are unkind to PLWHA are usually ignorant about HIV. They may be afraid of catching HIV. Sometimes they blame the people with HIV for getting the disease. Often PLWHA experience stigma and discrimination.

What can you tell them which would help?

Did you know?

Stigma is when someone is seen as different and less good. Stigma leads to discrimination.

Discrimination is treating someone differently and unfairly because they are seen as different.

Activity 3

Imagine you are a person living with HIV.

1. How do you think other people might show stigma and discrimination?
2. How might this make you feel?
3. How might this affect your life?

Reflection

How can I show positive attitudes to PLWHA?

▶ Theme: Sexuality and Sexual Health

EATING AND FITNESS

1 Fruit and Vegetables

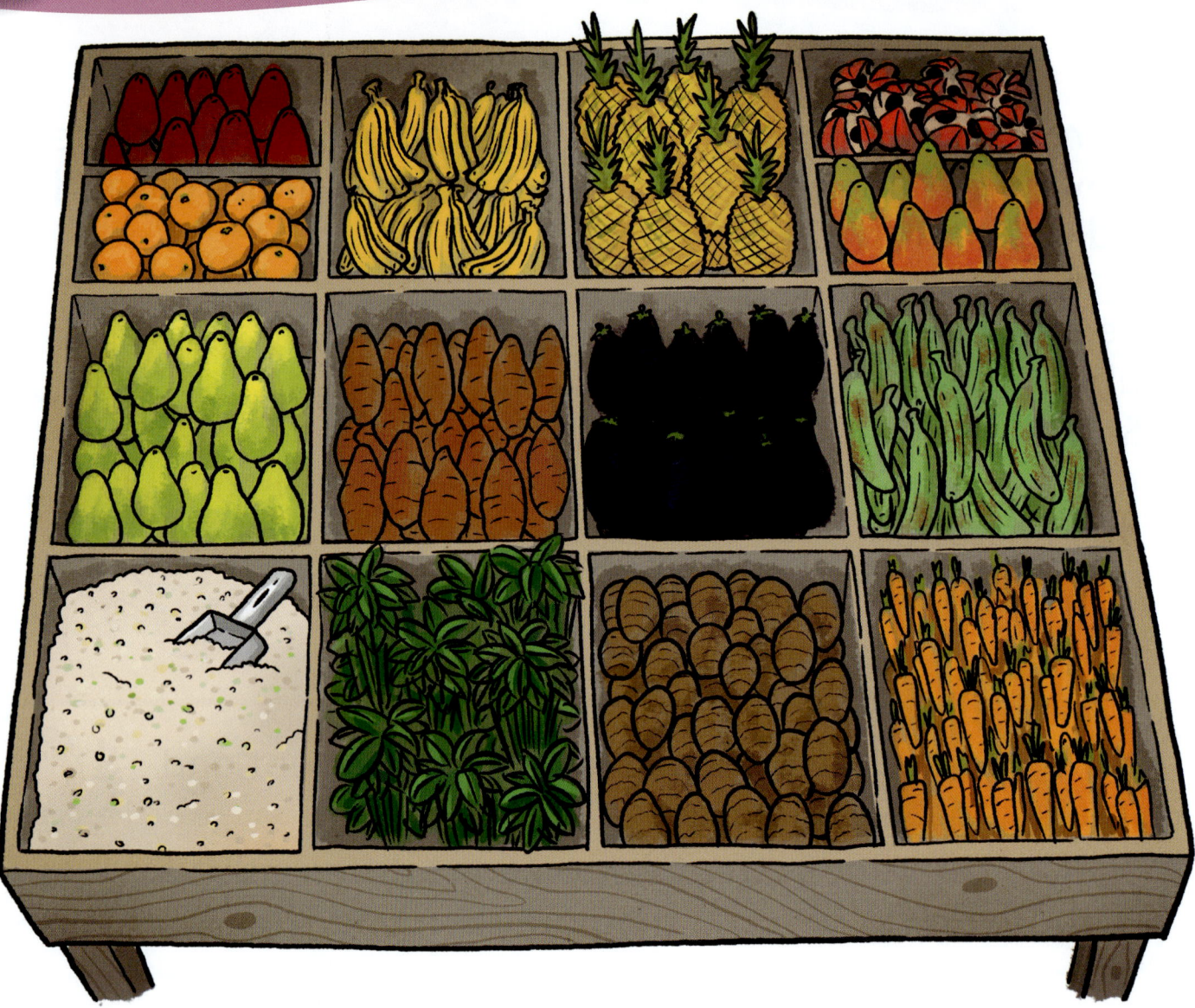

Activity 1

With your partner:
1 Name the fruits and vegetables you can see in the picture.
2 Pick your favourite fruit and your favourite vegetable. Tell your partner why you like to eat them.
3 Tell the class which fruit and vegetable are your partner's favourites and why.

Fruits and vegetables are very good for us. They contain:

- **carbohydrates**, which give us energy
- **fibre**, which helps our bodies use food and get rid of wastes
- **vitamins**, which help us grow and protect us from diseases
- **minerals**, which help us grow and protect us from diseases.

They also contain small amounts of proteins and good fats. Different fruits and vegetables have different vitamins and minerals. So it is important to eat a wide variety. Fruits and vegetables are also low in salt, fat and calories. You should eat five portions of fruit and vegetables each day.

Activity 2

1. **Discuss with your partner:** How many fruits or vegetables did you eat yesterday?
2. Look again at the picture on page 38. Choose at least five different fruits or vegetables you would like to eat today.

Reflection

Am I eating enough fruit and vegetables?
How can I persuade my family to eat more?

▶ Theme: Eating and Fitness

EATING AND FITNESS

Healthy Food Choices

In order to be healthy we need to eat a balanced diet. This means eating different kinds of foods: carbohydrates, fruits and vegetables, proteins and fats.

We need to eat:
- some of each kind of food every day
- more of some foods and less of others
- the right amount of foods.

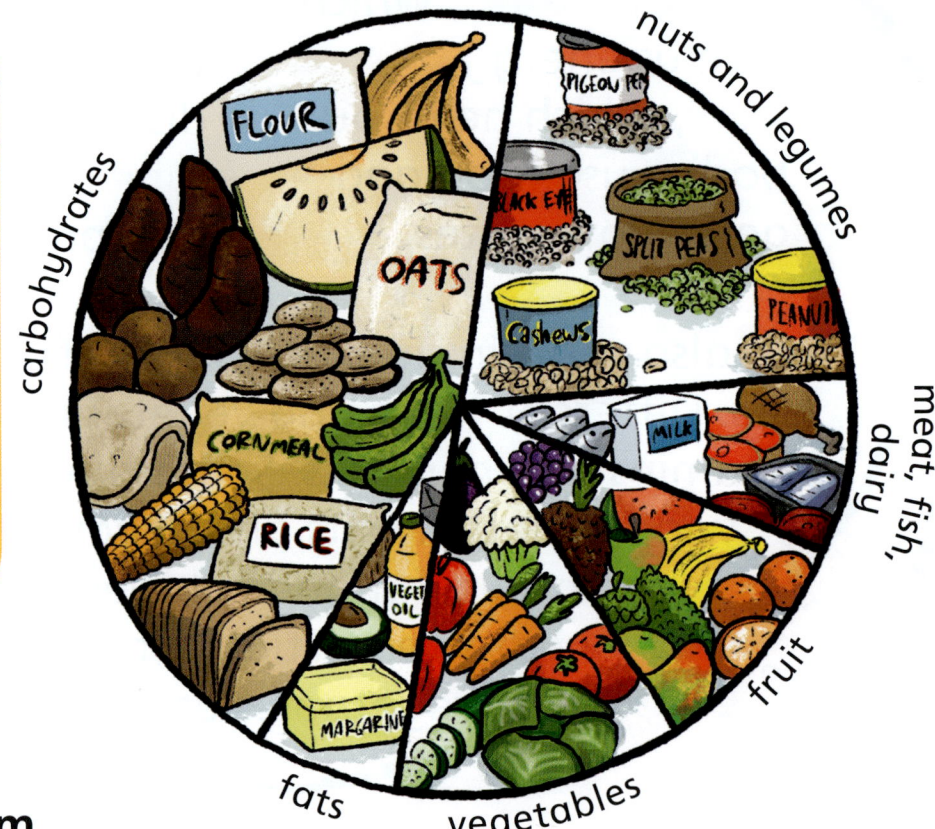

Activity 1

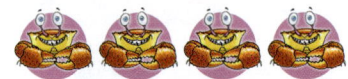

Look at the diagram.
1. What kind of foods should we eat most of? And the least?
2. Name some foods in each of the following groups: fats, proteins, fruit and vegetables, carbohydrates.

On Tuesday Rebecca ate and drank a banana and some milk for breakfast, a packet of chips with a cola at lunch-time, and she had some sweets on the way home from school. In the evening she ate a beef burger in a bun and a small amount of salad with mayonnaise and had another cola.

▶ Key Life Skills: **Critical thinking**, Decision-making, Healthy self-management

On Wednesday Rebecca ate a banana and orange for breakfast with some milk. At lunchtime she had a wholegrain sandwich with ham and salad in it, with orange juice. In the evening she had roast chicken with spinach, carrots and boiled sweet potatoes, followed by a mango.

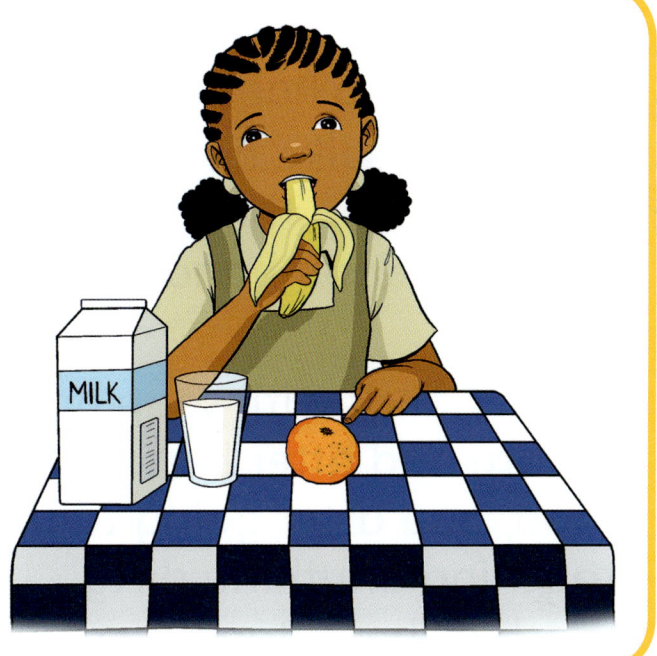

Activity 2

With your partner, talk about:
1 Which day did Rebecca eat a balanced diet?
2 Which meal was a healthy choice on both days?
3 Count and compare the number of fruit and vegetable portions on each day.
4 Which foods did Rebecca eat which are high in salt and fat?
5 Which of Rebecca's meals would you like to eat? Why?

Reflection

Do I eat a balanced diet? Are my meal choices healthy? What changes do I need to make?

EATING AND FITNESS

3 Safe Food

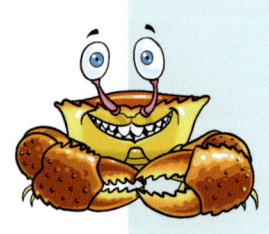

Germs can get onto our food and make us sick. We need to handle food safely.

Germs like dirty, wet and warm places. To kill them and stop them from multiplying we need to follow safe food-handling steps:

Clean

- Wash hands with soap and water before and after handling or eating food, and after going to the toilet or touching anything dirty.
- Wash dishes, utensils, cutting boards and kitchen surfaces with hot soapy water.
- Rinse fresh fruits and vegetables under running tap water.

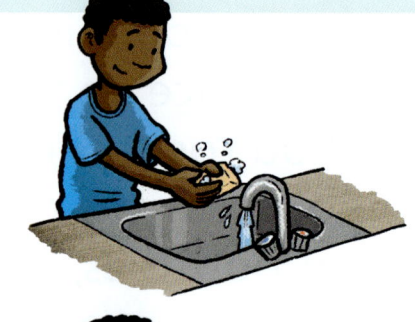

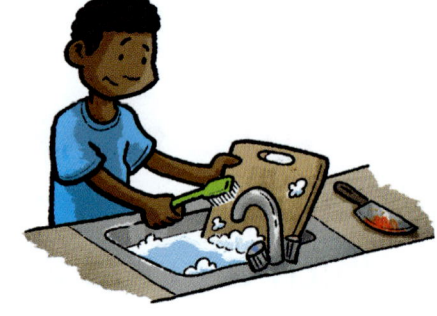

Separate

So that bacteria does not move onto other foods:

- Keep raw meat, seafood and eggs separate in bags and in the fridge.
- Use one chopping board for fresh vegetables and fruit and another for raw meat, poultry and seafood.

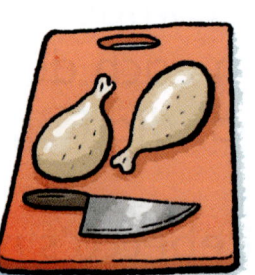 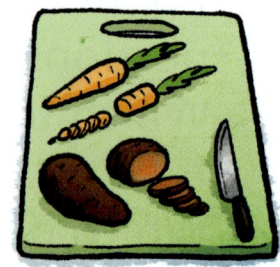

Cook

- Meat, eggs and fish should be cooked thoroughly to kill the germs.

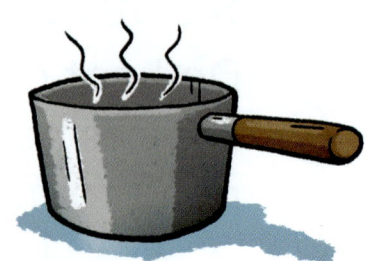

Chill

Cold stops germs from multiplying, so:
- put foods bought cold quickly into fridge or freezer
- do not leave raw meat, fish, eggs, cooked food or cut fruit and vegetables out of the fridge.

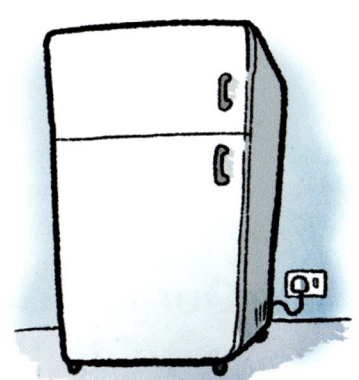

Activity 1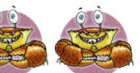

With your partner:
1. Decide on a meal you would like to cook together.
2. On separate pieces of paper or card, draw big pictures of foods for your meal (for example a chicken, rice, vegetables and fruit).
3. Role-play preparing and cooking your foods. Use the safe food handling steps above. Start from when you first go into the kitchen.
4. Write a list of the things you did.

> **Did you know?**
> One single germ can multiply into 8 million germs in 24 hours!

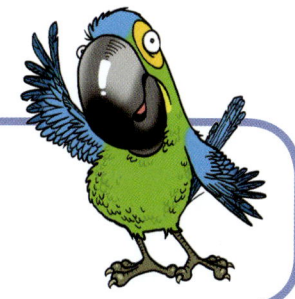

Activity 2

Make a poster about safe food handling to take home. Ask your family if you can put it up in the kitchen.

Reflection
How can we improve our food handling at home?

▶ Theme: Eating and Fitness

EATING AND FITNESS

4 Muscles and Movement

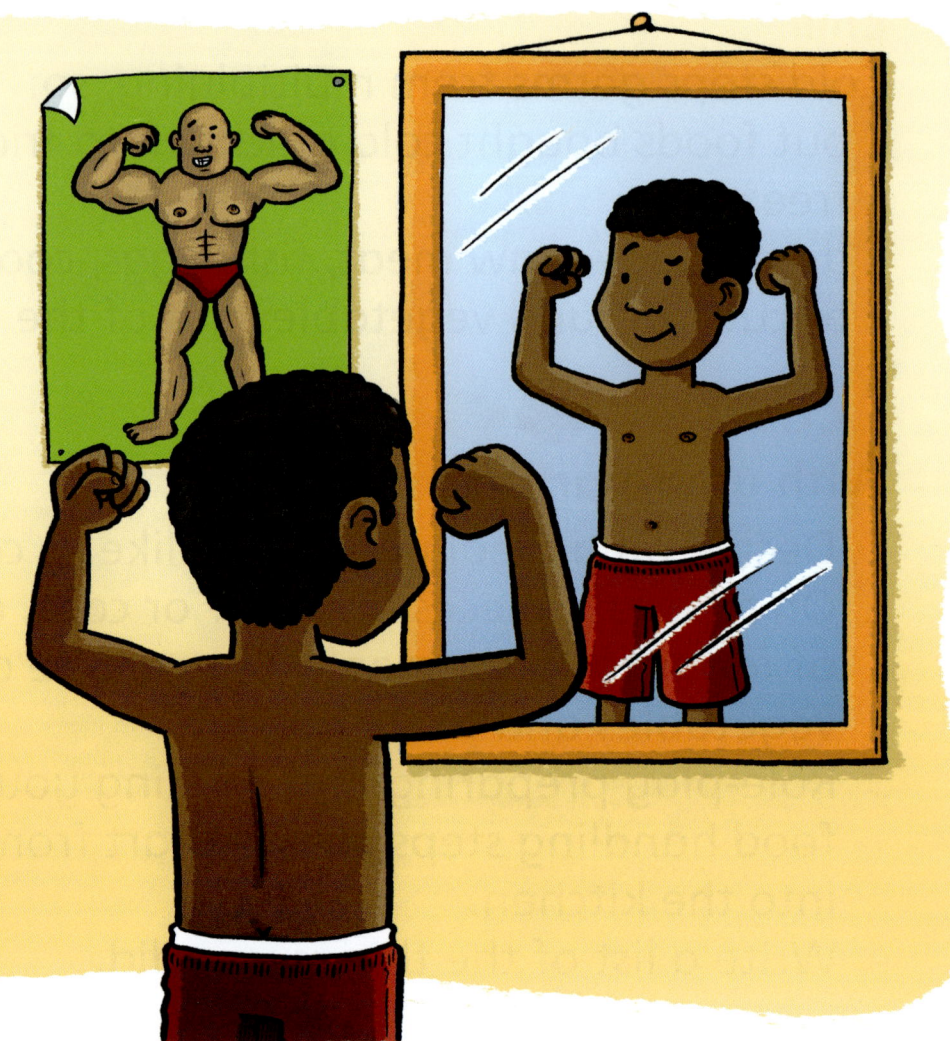

Our muscles help us to do things and to move. For healthy strong muscles we need to eat healthy foods, especially proteins, and exercise our muscles.

Activity 1

1 Move (bend) one arm at the elbow to lift a book up to your shoulder. With the other hand feel the muscle in the top of your arm working as you do this.

2 Now move the arm back down and feel the muscle behind your arm.

3 Try some exercises to work your muscles: sit-ups, press-ups, running on the spot, jumping on the spot.

▶ Key Life Skills: **Healthy self-management**, Critical thinking, Decision-making

Motor movements are the movements we make using our muscles.

Gross motor movements are big movements, like running, lifting something heavy or jumping.

Fine motor movements are small movements, like picking something up between your thumb and forefinger, or wiggling your toes.

To develop our muscles and physical skills we need to practise both kinds of movements.

Activity 2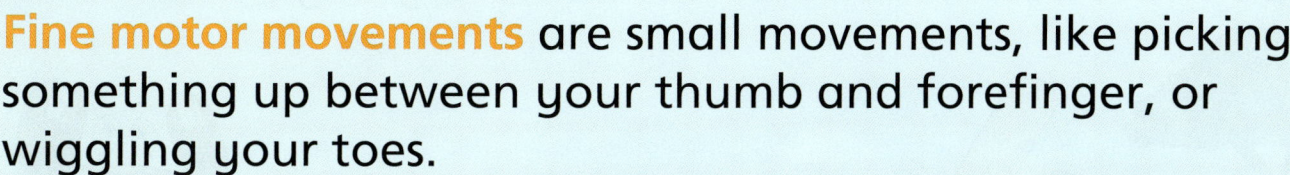

1. **Think of some fine motor movements you can do.**
2. **Practise them with your partner.**

Now share them with the class.

Reflection

Which of my muscles are stronger and which are weaker? What can I do to make the weaker muscles stronger? Which fine motor movements do I need to practise?

▶ Theme: Eating and Fitness

EATING AND FITNESS

5 Safe Exercise and Competition

For healthy living we need to work, play, exercise and rest.

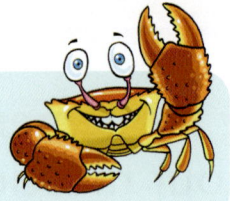

Physical exercise is good for us. It strengthens our muscles, and our heart and lungs. It gives us energy and helps us to cope with stress. We should exercise every day.

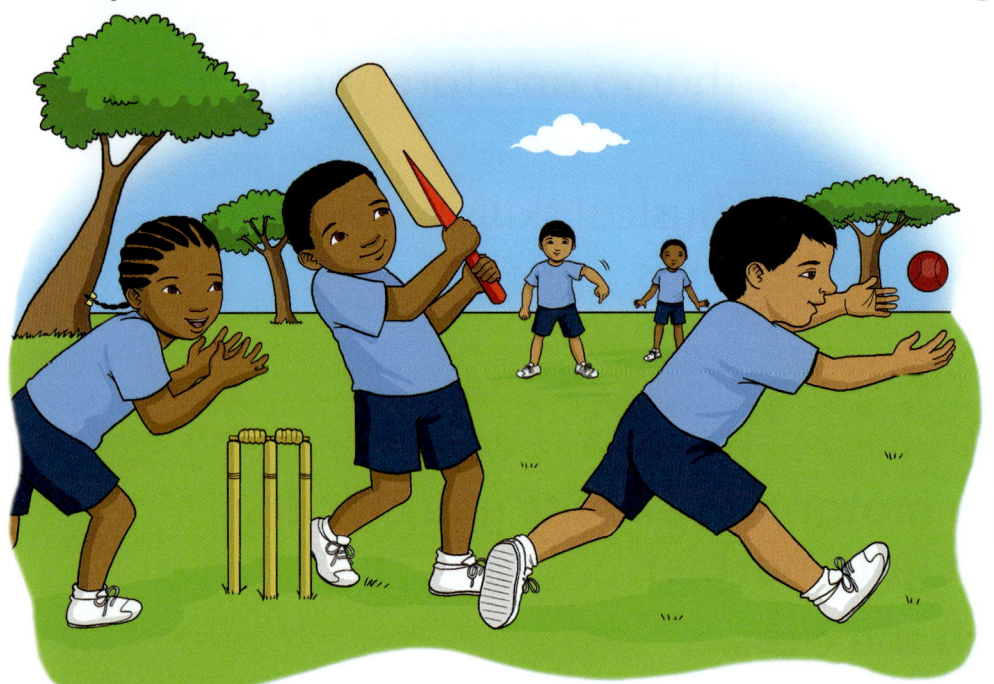

When we exercise or do physical activity we must do it safely.

Activity 1

Talk about the physical activities you do.
1. Why are they good for you?
2. Which ones do you dislike and why?
3. Which ones do you enjoy and why?

Activity 2

Choose one physical sport or game you play.
1. What safety rules are there?
2. Choose one rule and explain how it keeps you safe.

▶ Key Life Skills: **Healthy self-management,** Communication, Critical thinking

Activity 3

Discuss as a class:
1. What do we like about playing in teams?
2. What do we dislike?
3. How does playing in teams help you?

Often we play in teams. This helps us to learn to work together and improve our communication skills.

When we do sports, we often compete with other people. This can be stressful. Get plenty of sleep, train well, eat healthily, and talk with your coach and team mates.

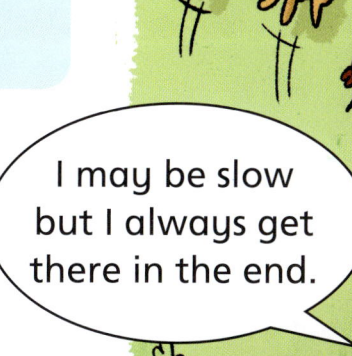

Activity 4

Talk about competing at sports.
1. How do you feel before you compete?
2. How do you feel when you win?
3. How do you feel when you lose?
4. How do you express these feelings?

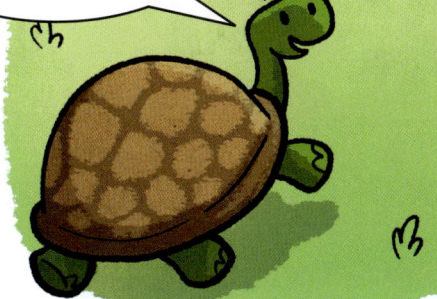

I may be slow but I always get there in the end.

Reflection

Do I pay attention to safety when doing physical activities? How can I improve safety?

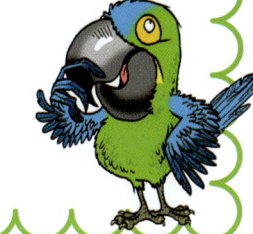

▶ Theme: Eating and Fitness

EATING AND FITNESS

Eating and Fitness Choices

What we eat and our fitness is affected by:
- our age
- our health
- our food and exercise needs
- our family habits.

What we eat is also affected by our ethnicity, religion and community.

Can you think of any other things which affect our eating and fitness choices?

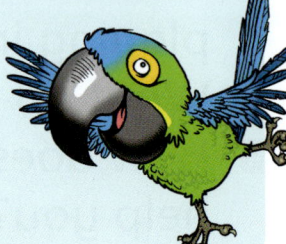

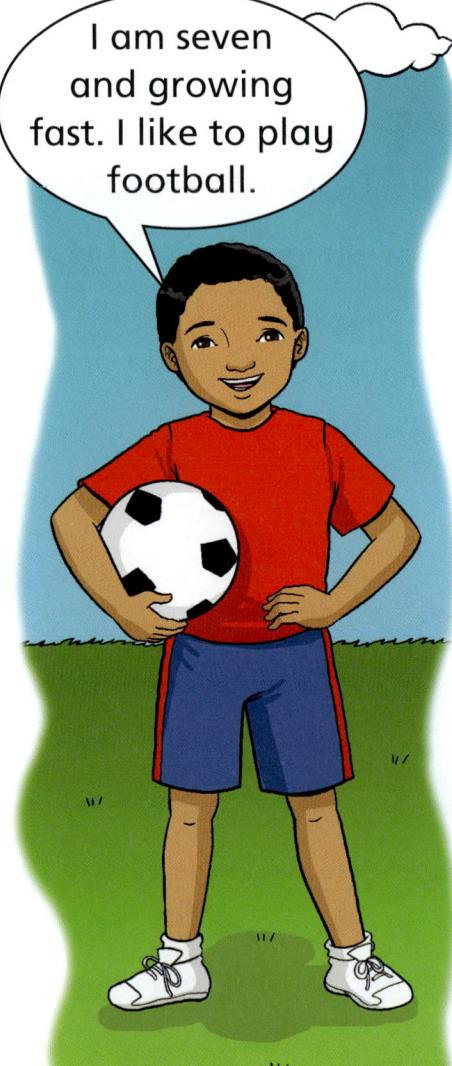

I am seven and growing fast. I like to play football.

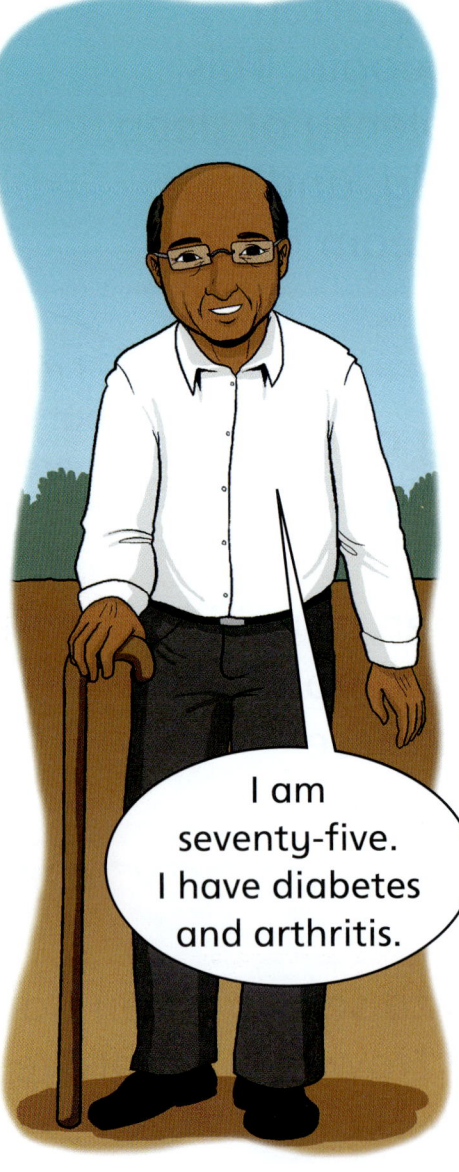

I am seventy-five. I have diabetes and arthritis.

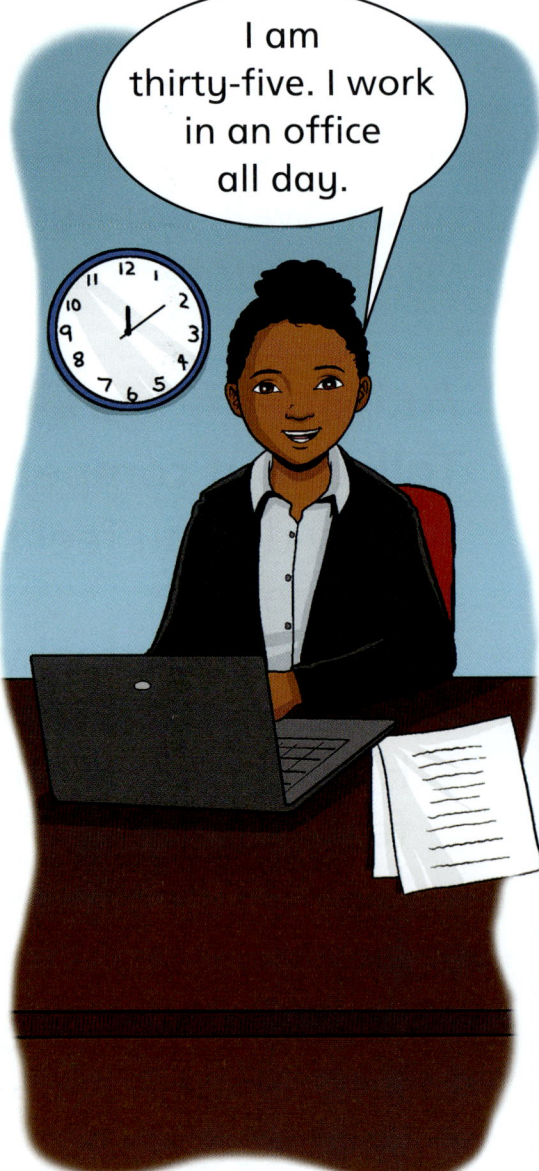

I am thirty-five. I work in an office all day.

▶ Key Life Skills: **Critical thinking**, Communication, Self-awareness

Activity 1

In groups, choose ONE of the people in the pictures. Talk about:

1. How old are they?
2. How healthy are they?
3. How much physical exercise do you think they do?
4. Name some foods you think they might like to eat.

Share your ideas with the class.

Activity 2

With your partner, talk about:

1. How do your own age and health affect the food you eat?
2. How does the amount of physical activity you do affect the amount of food you need?
3. How do your family habits and ethnic group affect the foods you eat?
4. Do your religious beliefs affect the food you eat?

Share your ideas with the class.

Reflection

What factors affect my food choices? What factors affect my physical activity? Do I do enough physical activity?

▶ Theme: Eating and Fitness

MANAGING THE ENVIRONMENT

1 Our Environment

Our **environment** is everything around us. We can divide it into **natural** and **built** (human-made) things. Human beings change the environment.

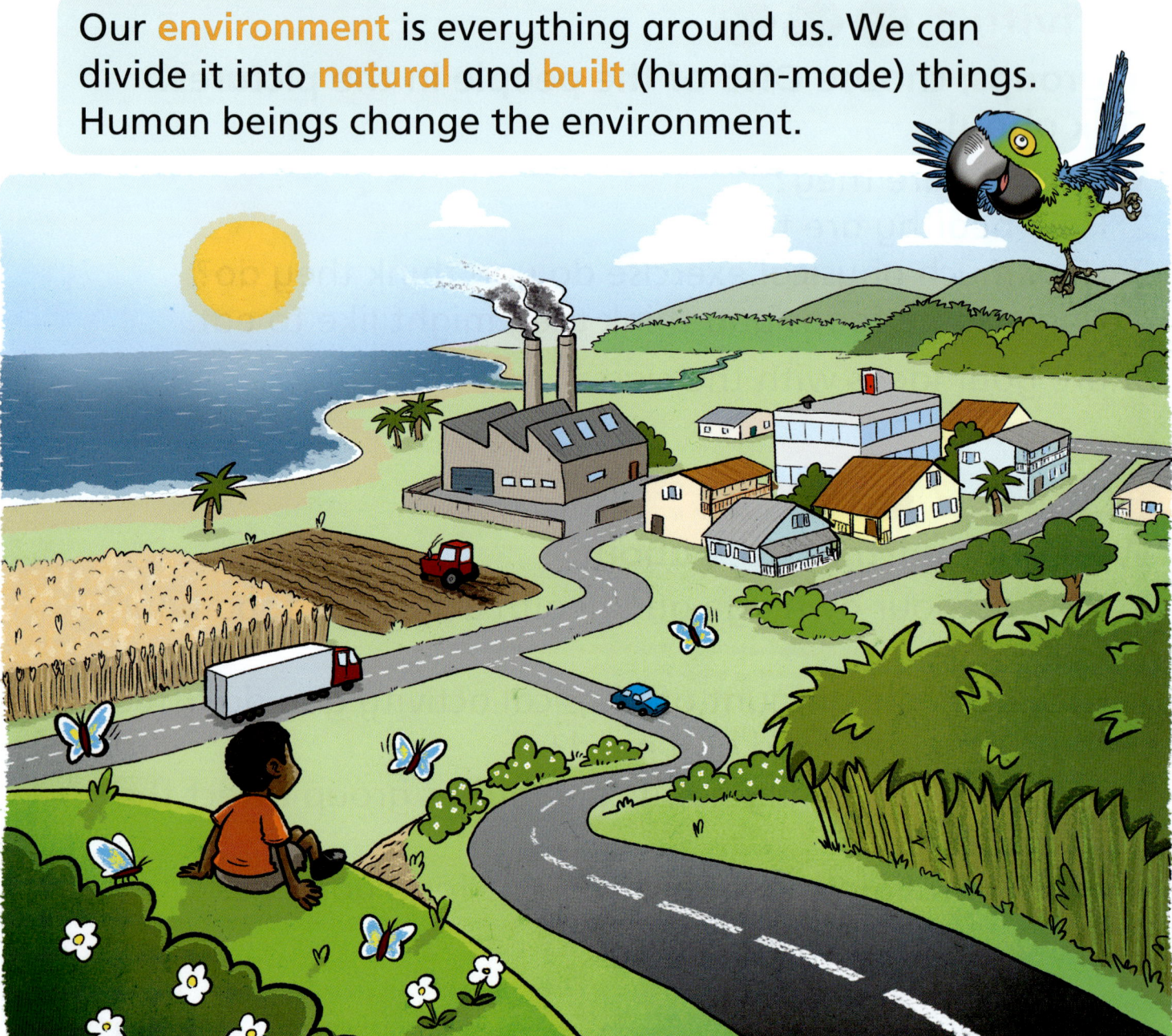

Activity 1

Look at the picture with your partner. Find:
1 four natural things
2 four built or human-made things
3 two ways in which humans have changed the natural environment.

50 ▶ Key Life Skills: **Critical thinking**, Communication, Self-monitoring

Did you know?

Our natural environment has different parts:
- **Non-living things**: air, water, sunlight, land.
- **Living things**: plants, animals and humans.

These all depend on each other. They are balanced. When humans change one part, this affects all the other parts.

Activity 2

1. **Think of at least one way in which we use each part of the environment.**
2. **Think of one way humans change part of the environment. How does this affect other parts?**

We call the natural things that we use **natural resources**. There is a limit to the amounts of natural resources in our environment. If we use too much of a resource or damage it then it can run out.

Reflection

How do I affect the natural environment? How can I protect the natural environment?

▶ Theme: Managing the Environment

MANAGING THE ENVIRONMENT

2 Trees and Forests

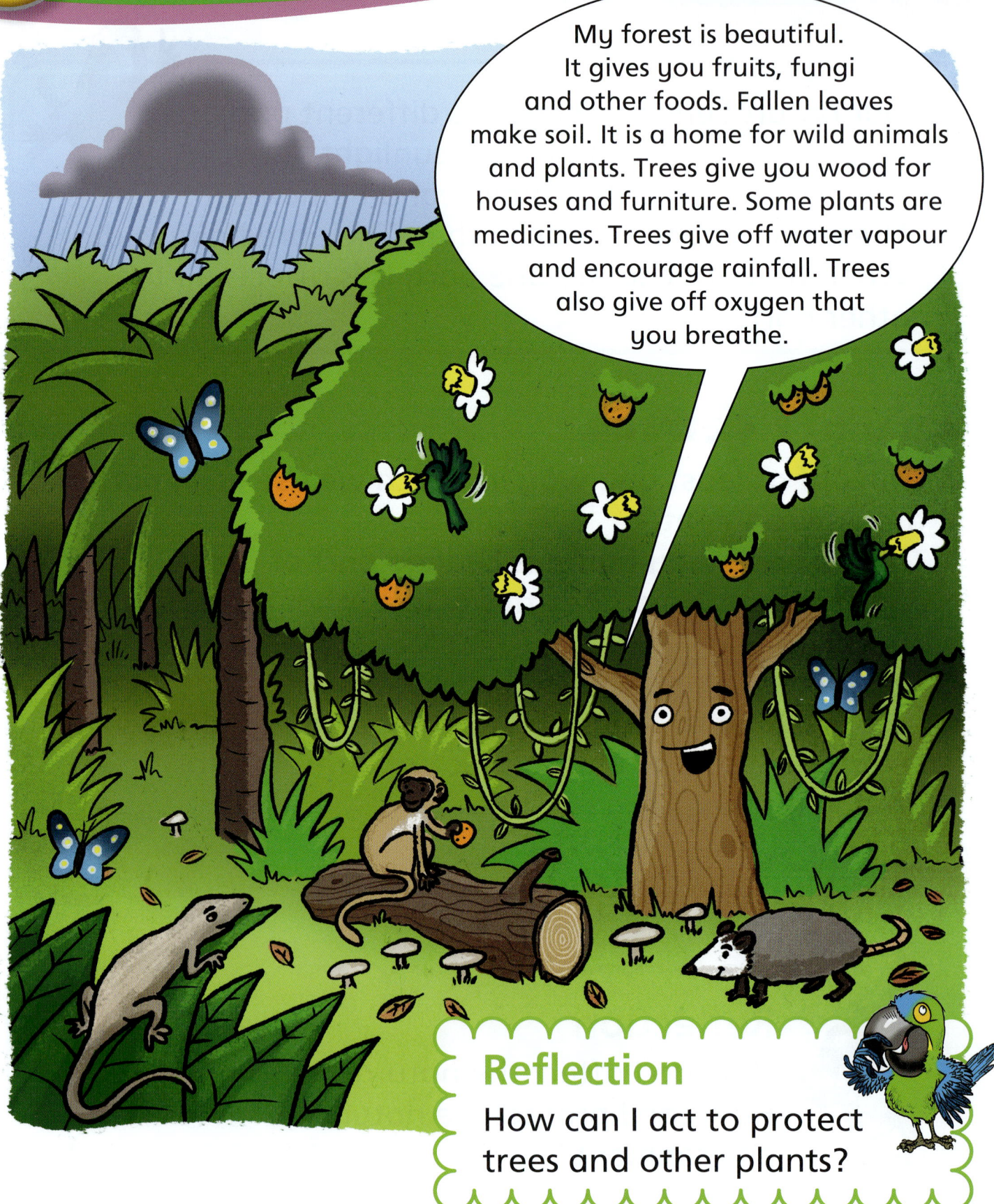

My forest is beautiful. It gives you fruits, fungi and other foods. Fallen leaves make soil. It is a home for wild animals and plants. Trees give you wood for houses and furniture. Some plants are medicines. Trees give off water vapour and encourage rainfall. Trees also give off oxygen that you breathe.

Reflection

How can I act to protect trees and other plants?

Key Life Skills: **Problem-solving**, Communication, Self-monitoring

Activity 1

Look at the picture with your partner.
1. In what ways is the forest useful to us?
2. What happens when we cut forests down?

Share your ideas with the class.

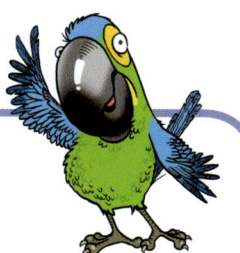

> **Did you know?**
> Paper is made from trees. One tree will make about 100 books like this one.

Activity 2

1. **Name some of the plants that you eat.**
2. **Name some other ways you use plants.**
3. **How else are plants important?**

In some places forests and other plants are being destroyed. Forests are cut down for timber and to provide farm land. Mangroves and swamps are removed to build hotels and other buildings. Grasslands are overgrazed by putting too many cows to feed on them.

Activity 3

1. **Say how plants help to make a healthy environment.**
2. **Suggest some ways you can care for forests and other plants.**

▶ Theme: Managing the Environment

MANAGING THE ENVIRONMENT

3 Pollution

When harmful materials go into the environment we call this **pollution**. Pollution is caused by many different human activities. It affects our land, air and water.

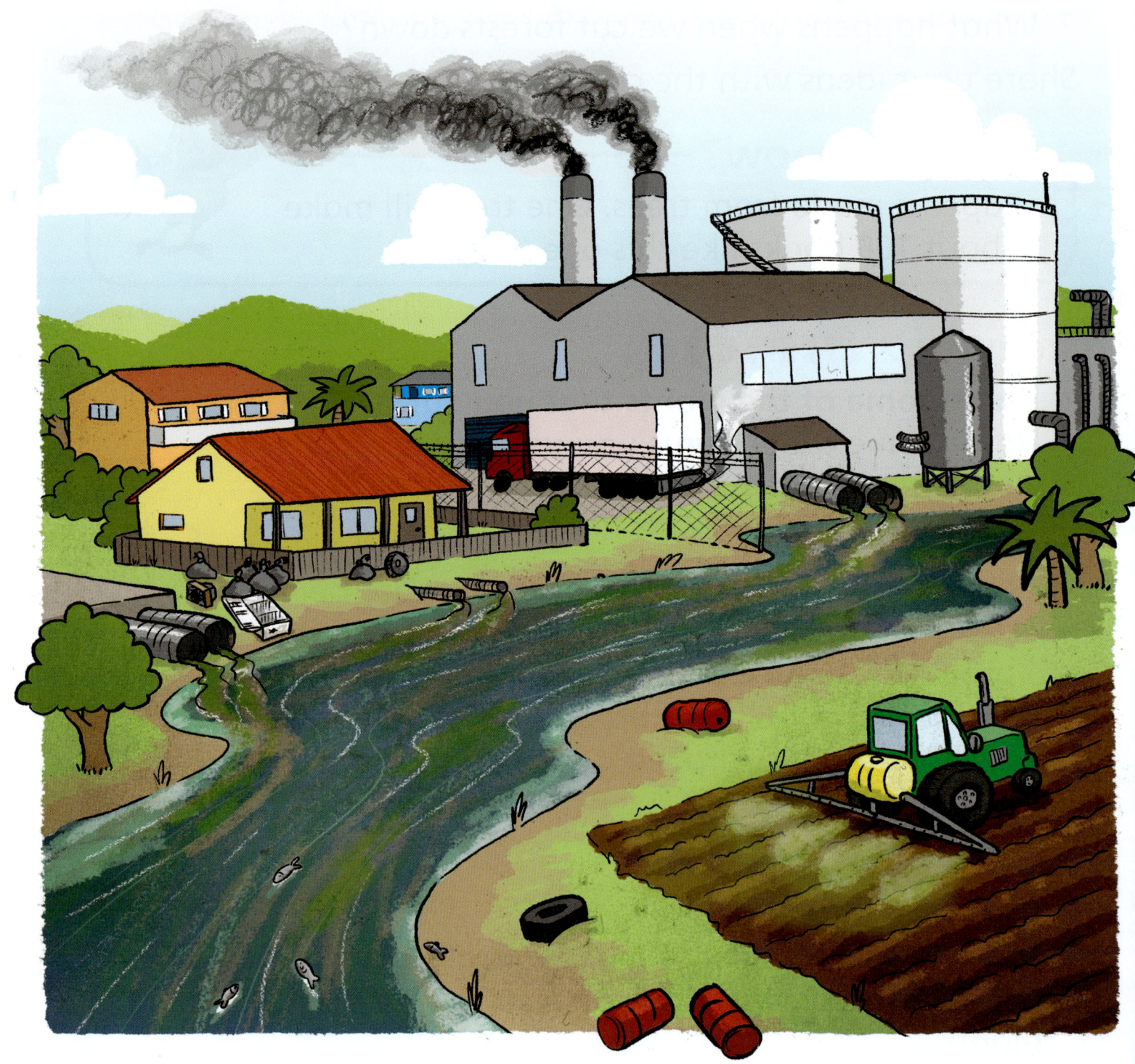

54 ▶ Key Life Skills: **Problem-solving**, Communication, Healthy self-management

Activity 1

Look at the picture with your partner.

1. Name two ways in which air is being polluted.
2. Name two ways in which water is being polluted.
3. Name two ways in which land is being polluted.

Activity 2

Talk about pollution in your community or country.

1. What is it caused by?
2. How does it affect us?
3. What can we do about it?

Pollution can make us ill:

- Air pollution causes asthma and other breathing problems.
- Water pollution causes stomach illnesses such as diarrhoea.
- Land pollution, such as throwing garbage in gullies, spreads disease.

Did you know?

Smoking pollutes the air and causes illnesses for the smoker and those around.

Reflection

Does anything I do cause pollution? What can I do to stop polluting the environment?

▶ Theme: Managing the Environment

MANAGING THE ENVIRONMENT

4 Put It in the Bin!

What do we do with our garbage at school?
What do we do with our garbage at home?
We put it in the bin!

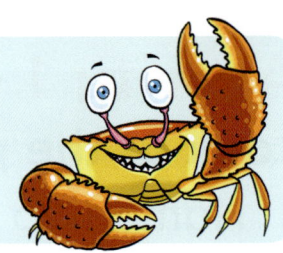

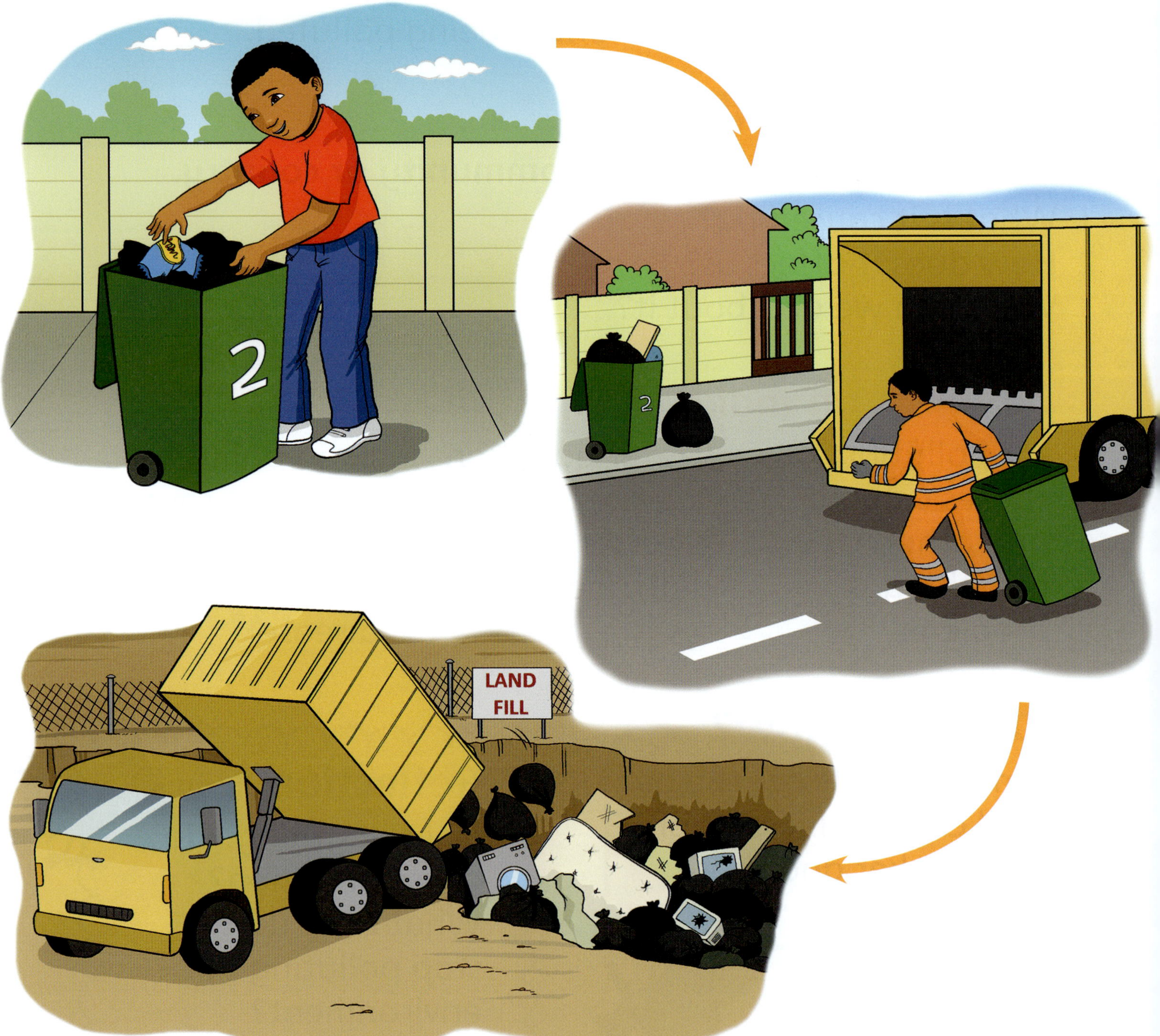

Key Life Skills: **Advocacy,** Communication, Healthy self-management

Activity 1

With your partner, explain:
1. What's happening in the pictures.
2. Where our garbage ends up.

> **Did you know?**
> Rats, mice, flies and mosquitoes spread diseases. Garbage and litter attract rats, mice and flies. They feed on the garbage.
> Pools of water attract mosquitoes and other insects.

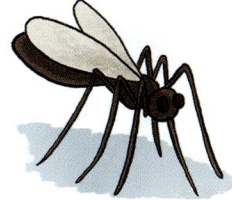 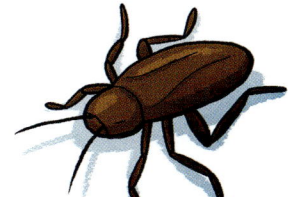 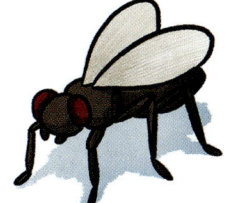 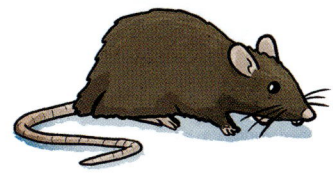

Activity 2

Talk about the following in small groups.
1. Which animals carry diseases?
2. What can we do to make our environment healthier at school and home?
3. Together create a song about making a healthier environment.

> **Reflection**
> Do I always put my garbage in the bin?

▶ Theme: Managing the Environment

MANAGING THE ENVIRONMENT

5 Improving Our Environment

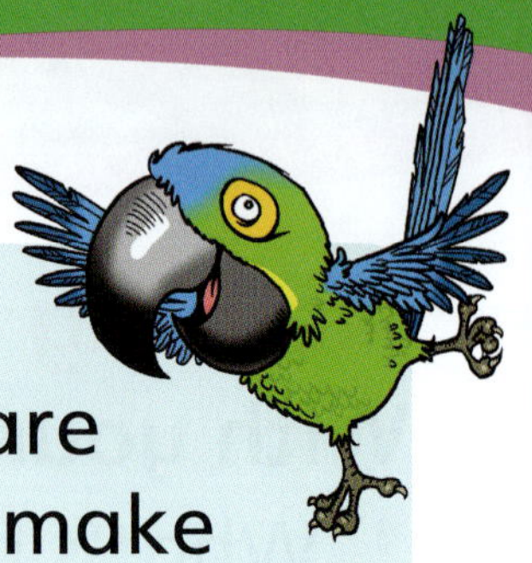

A clean environment is a healthy environment. The children in Grade 2 at Hummingbird School are environmental monitors. They take it in turns to make sure the school is clean and safe.

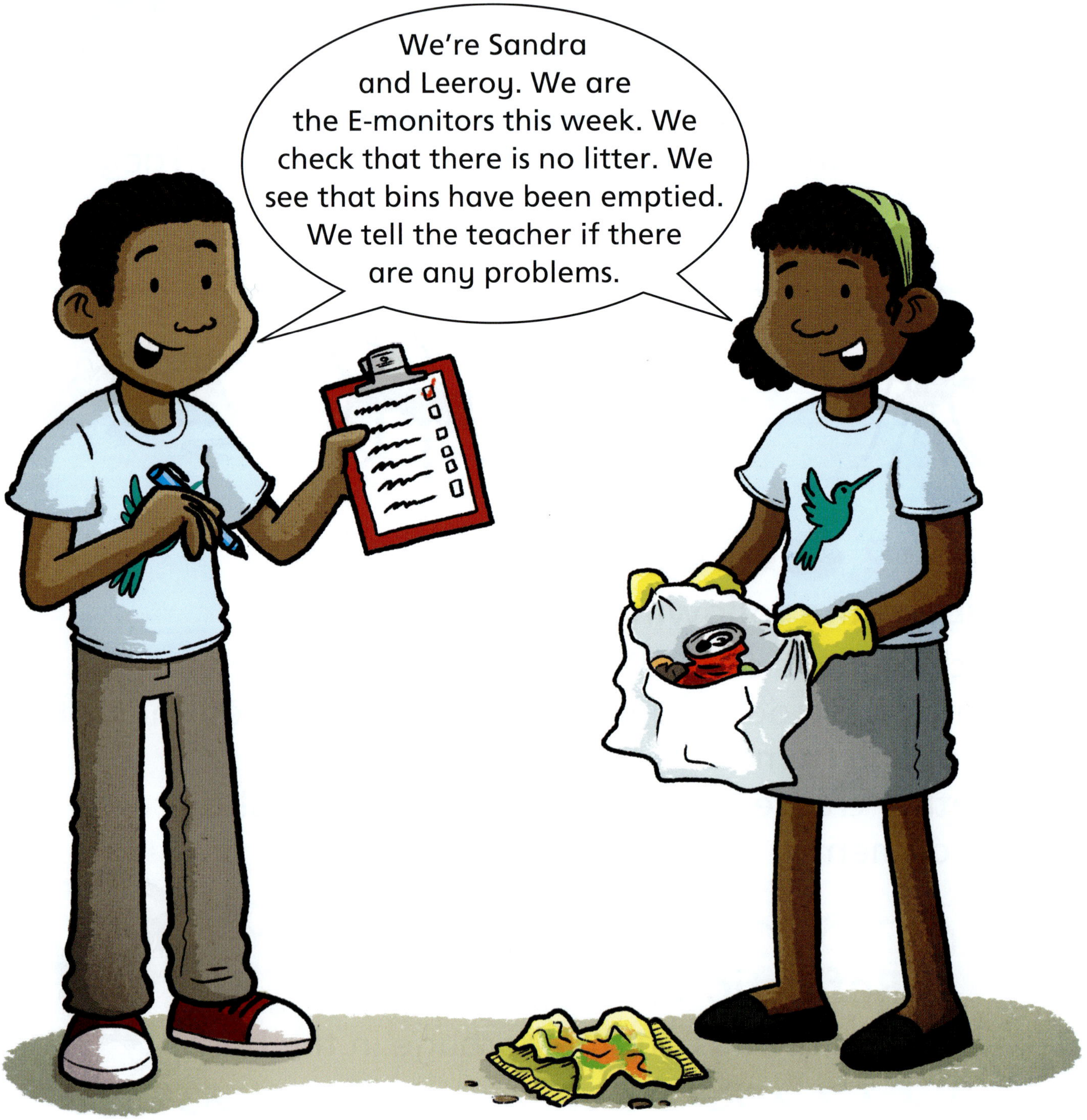

> We're Sandra and Leeroy. We are the E-monitors this week. We check that there is no litter. We see that bins have been emptied. We tell the teacher if there are any problems.

Key Life Skills: **Creative thinking,** Advocacy, Self-monitoring

Activity 1

Get into groups. From what you have learnt already, suggest some ways you can make your school environment clean and healthy:

- in the classroom
- in the school building
- in the playground.

Share your ideas with the class.

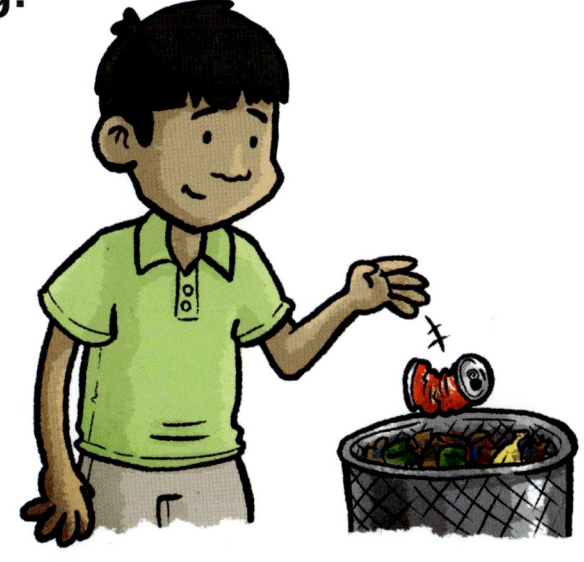

Activity 2

1. With your partner, write a list of tasks a class E-monitor could do.
2. Talk about whether each class member should be E-monitor for one day or one week.
3. How many children should be E-monitors at one time?

Share your ideas with the class.

Reflection

What can I do to improve my environment at home?

▶ Theme: Managing the Environment

MANAGING THE ENVIRONMENT

6 Reduce, Reuse, Recycle

We all throw away too many things and make too much waste. The landfill sites where we put our garbage are filling up and we don't have much land for new ones. Also, we are using up the Earth's resources, such as forests and oil.

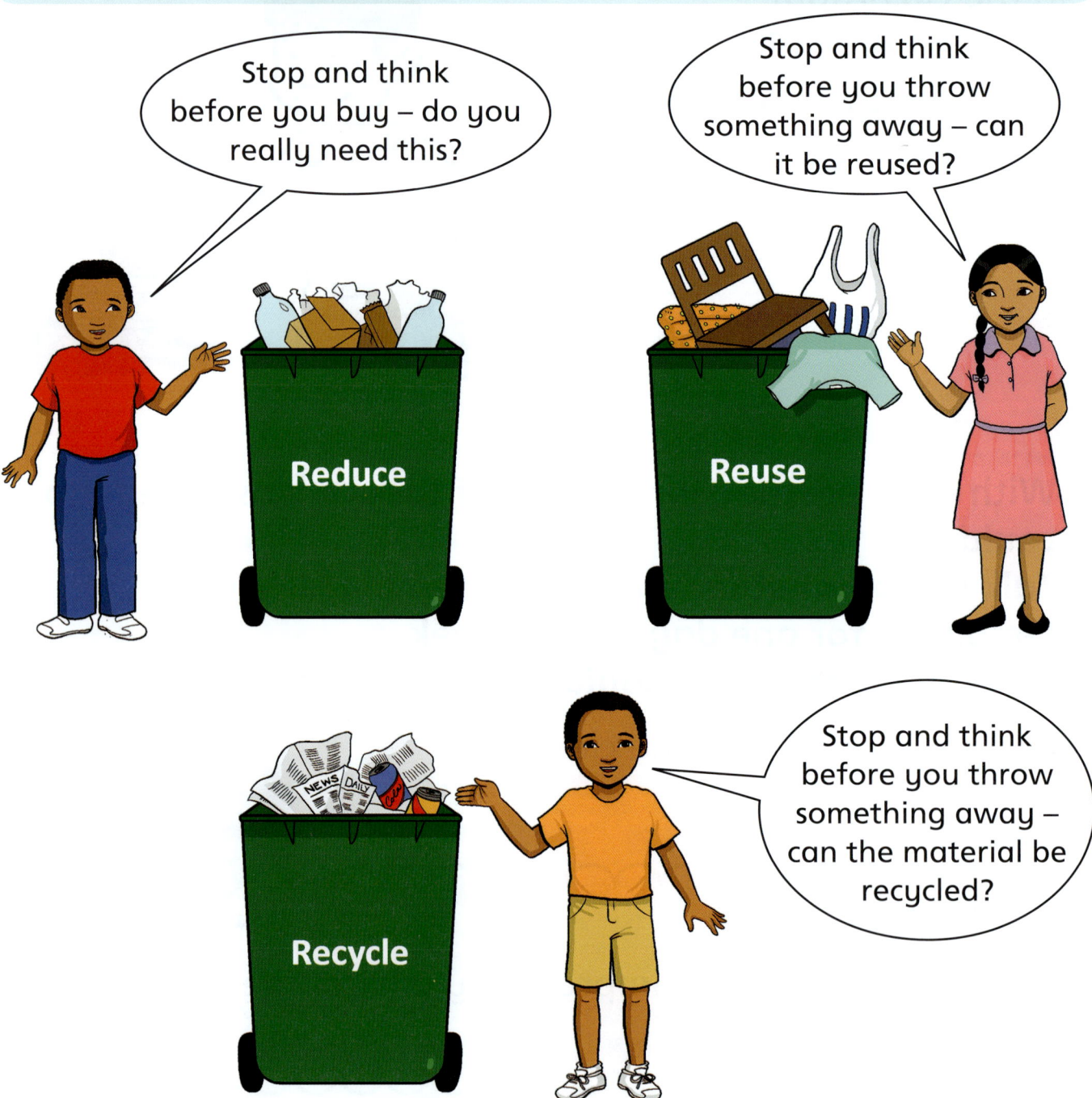

Stop and think before you buy – do you really need this?

Reduce

Stop and think before you throw something away – can it be reused?

Reuse

Stop and think before you throw something away – can the material be recycled?

Recycle

▶ Key Life Skills: **Critical thinking,** Communication, Healthy self-management

The 3 Rs

Reduce: means we use fewer resources and produce less waste. We can buy less and avoid lots of packaging.

Reuse: means we use things again and again, or we pass them to other people to reuse.

Recycle: means we reuse the material and make it into something else.

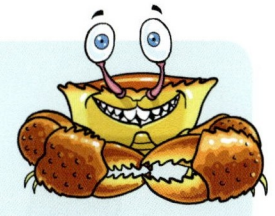

Activity 1

In your group, talk about:
1 Something you or a family member bought which you didn't really need.
2 Something which can be reused instead of thrown away.
3 Something that can be recycled. Share your ideas with the class.

Activity 2

Make a classroom display of three bins: Reduce, Reuse, Recycle with pictures of things that can go into each.

Reflection
How can I reduce, reuse and recycle to protect the environment?

▶ Theme: Managing the Environment

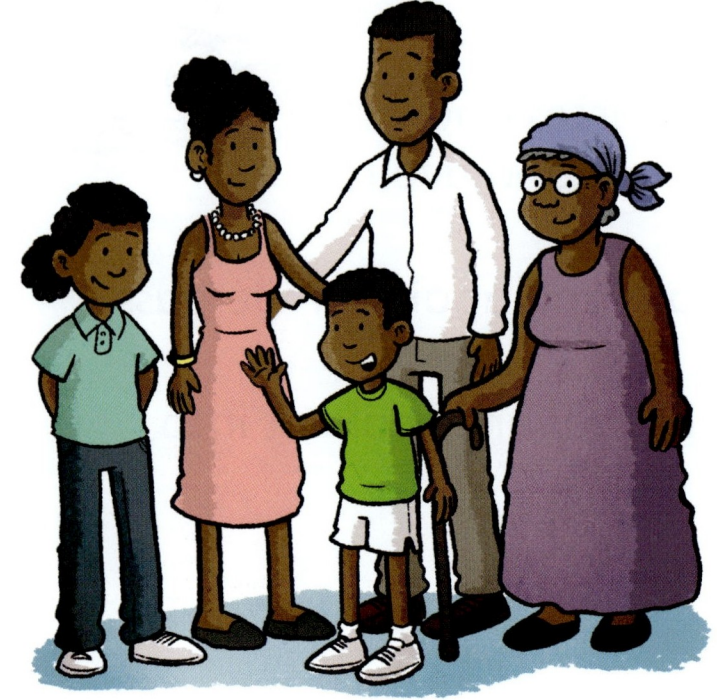
family

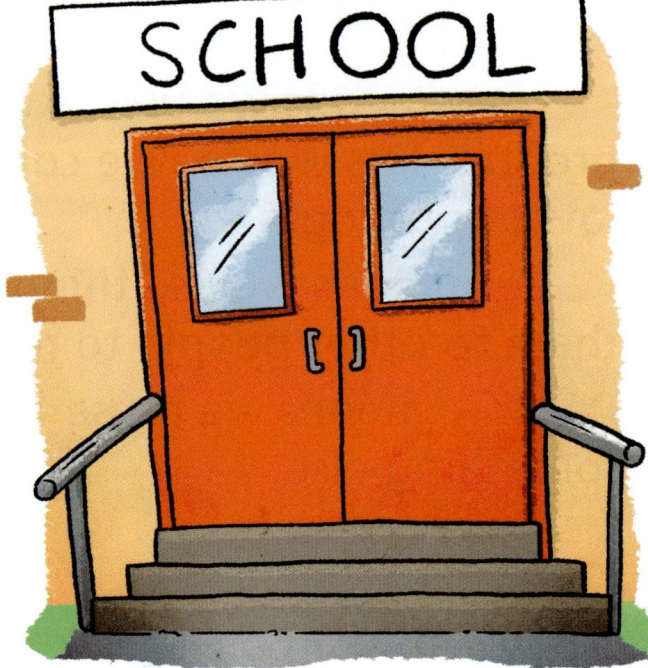
school

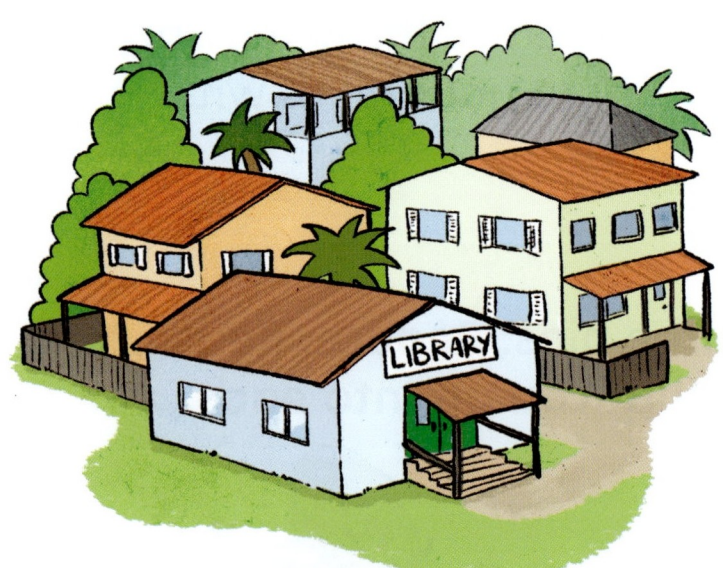
community

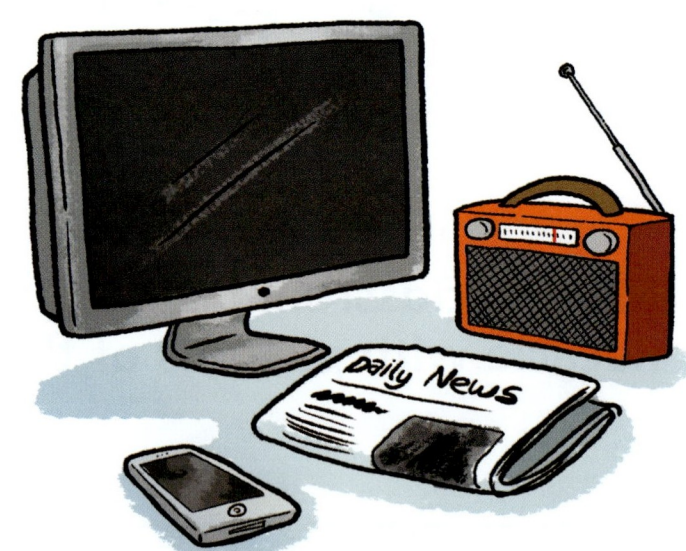
media

When we learn about the environment we need to find things out. We can use the sources above.

Key Life Skills: **Communication**, Decision-making, Healthy self-management

Activity 1

1 **With your partner, talk about who you could ask about the environment:**
   - at home, in the family
   - at school
   - in the community or neighbourhood.

2 **Which media sources might be able to help you?**

> You could find out more about the environment from organisations such as UNEP (the United Nations Environmental Programme), Earthwatch or World Wide Fund for Nature. Your teacher will help you.

Activity 2

Now think back over what you have learnt this year in the other three themes: Self and Interpersonal Relationships, Sexuality and Sexual Health and Eating and Fitness.

1 In groups choose one of the other three themes. Who could you ask to find out more:
   - at home?
   - at school?
   - in the community?

2 Which media sources could you use?

Reflection
What is the most important thing I have learnt in HFLE this year?

▶ Theme: Managing the Environment

Macmillan Education
4 Crinan Street, London, N1 9XW
A division of Macmillan Education Limited

Companies and representatives throughout the world.

www.macmillan-caribbean.com

ISBN: 9780-230-43175-1

Text © Clare Eastland 2015
Design and illustration © Macmillan Education Limited 2015

The author has asserted her rights to be identified as the author of this work in accordance with the Copyright, Design and Patents Act 1988.

First published 2015

All rights reserved; no part of this publication may be reproduced, stored in a retrieval system, transmitted in any form, or by any means, electronic, mechanical, photocopying, recording, or otherwise, without the prior written permission of the publishers.

Designed by Macmillan Education
Illustrated by Tamara Joubert and Joseph Wilkins
Cover design by Andrew Magee Design Ltd
Cover photograph courtesy of Corbis / Mother Image / Benjamin A. Paterson (front)
Cover illustration by Mark Draisey
Layout and typesetting by Jim Weaver

The publishers and author team would like to thank Fortuna Anthony, Jenelle Babb, Hermione Baptiste, Vindra Cassie, Gerard Drakes, Elaine King, Glenda Rolle, Rebecca Tortello, Esther Utoh and Pat Warner for their invaluable help and advice at every stage of this series.

These materials may contain links for third party websites. We have no control over, and are not responsible for, the contents of such third party websites. Please use care when accessing them. Although we have tried to trace and contact copyright holders before publication, in some cases this has not been possible. If contacted we will be pleased to rectify any errors or omissions at the earliest opportunity.

Printed and bound in Great Britain by Bell and Bain Ltd, Glasgow
2021
10 9 8 7